COLLINS GEM
CATS

a mine of information

C000077247

COLLINS GEM
HORSES
& PONIES

a mine of information

INSECTS

KINGS &
QUEENS

MUSHROOMS
& TOADSTOOLS

COLLINS GEM
SNAKES

a mine of information

COLLINS GEM
SPIDERS

a mine of information

COLLINS GEM
STRESS
Survival Guide

a mine of information

COLLINS GEM
TAROT

a mine of information

COLLINS GEM
WINE
Guide

a mine of information

COLLINS GEM
WORLD
atlas

a mine of information

COLLINS GEM
YOGA

a mine of information

COLLINS GEM
ZODIAC
Types

a mine of information

COLLINS GEM

Healthy
EATING

Karen Sullivan

HarperCollins*Publishers*

Karen Sullivan has written over 20 books on health, nutrition and complementary medicine. She also lectures widely on women's health and other health issues.

HarperCollins Publishers
PO Box, Glasgow G4 0NB

Created and produced by
Grapevine Publishing Services, London

First published 1999

Reprint 10 9 8 7 6 5 4 3 2 1 0

Photographs by Christina Jansen

ISBN 0 00 472322-8

Printed in Italy by Amadeus S.p.A.

Contents

Introduction

We live in an era when food has never been so plentiful.
We have more varieties of foods from across the globe,
readily available in our local supermarkets, than our
parents ever dreamed of. We have a range of new ways
to cook our foods: the advent of microwaves has made

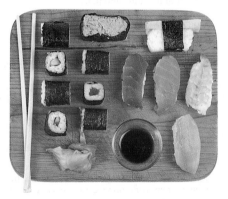

cooking all types of foods much quicker and more
efficient; we have adopted cooking methods, such as
stir-frying, from countries around the world; and we
have a variety of new implements, from food processors
and toasters through to grills and convection ovens, to
make preparation easier.

Why, then, are our eating habits so bad? The idea that a well-balanced diet, full of vitamins and minerals, is essential for a healthy body is nothing new. We know the message is getting through, because the sales of vitamin tablets have increased by over 200 percent in the last decade. But it seems that despite being more aware about the foods we should be eating, few of us actually put healthy eating into practice.

OUR MODERN LIFESTYLE

One of the factors affecting our choice of diet is the modern lifestyle. More and more families are dual earning, which means that both partners have little time for food shopping and preparation. Add to that the fact that fewer than 1 in 5 British families sit down and eat together and you have the makings of a culture in which 'mealtimes' as they were previously known are becoming increasingly irregular, and in some families, non-existent.

We try to fit too much into our lives, and food and mealtimes are falling lower and lower on our list of priorities. We eat on the run, grab a take-away on the journey home from work, pop a convenience food into the microwave and eat it in front of the television, and choose quick snacks in favour of well-balanced meals.

Food should be appreciated, shared and enjoyed. As parents, we must be careful not to feel guilty if children do not want what we think they should have. At the same time, they need to be offered nutritious food, and they need regular meals. Many of our eating habits stem from sharing mealtimes together. Children in particular learn social and cultural values during mealtimes, as well as getting nourishment.

We need to replan, making time for life's priorities – one of the most important of which is healthy eating. The whole business of eating and drinking should never be an afterthought. We are, quite simply, what we eat. Every mouthful, every supermarket expedition, every trip to the market, is your chance to become healthier and happier.

We don't yet know the long-term effects of living on a diet of TV dinners and refined foods because they have not been around long enough. However, there are indications that the health of ourselves and of our children is being seriously undermined by the modern diet of processed and chemically created foods.

WE ARE CHANGING THE WAY WE THINK

In the past we were willing to let the experts decide what food was good for us and our children. Now we are starting to question those experts. After 1945, great emphasis was placed on consuming sufficient milk, butter and meat. Recently there has been concern over the level of heart disease connected with a Western diet that is high in animal fats. If we are to believe the recent research, our Western diet is the root of hundreds of health problems, from cardio-vascular illness through to obesity.

But gradually, the message is getting through. More of us are choosing fresh, whole foods in favour of less nutritious options. Supermarkets are starting to stock a wide range of organic foods, and manufacturers are changing the way they prepare foods, with fewer unnatural ingredients and additives in their products.

WHO HAS TIME?

The idea of healthy eating is not a compelling one. Who needs to spend hours in the supermarket reading labels when you can buy something ready-made? Who wants to worry about getting enough vitamins when you can buy them in a bottle? Who has time to keep up to date with all the ever-changing information about food?

But eating healthily doesn't have to mean any of that. Once you've got to grips with the basics, you can concentrate on enjoying a delicious, nutritious diet that will leave you feeling better than you could ever have believed possible.

ENJOY YOUR FOOD!

Healthy food is full of flavour, colour and fresh, natural ingredients. Healthy food entices the senses,

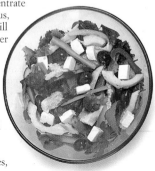

encourages you to enjoy what you are eating, and leaves you feeling satisfied. Most importantly, however, nutritious is delicious.

And a healthy diet can be much cheaper. Carefully selected, fresh foods are much less expensive than processed, ready-prepared meals, and new ways of cooking, including stir-frys, roasting and steaming, mean that food can be prepared quickly and nutritiously.

WHAT THIS BOOK CAN DO FOR YOU

This book focuses on what we need from our diet, and how to get it safely and effectively. All of the main issues involving our modern-day food are examined – from pesticides and food-borne illnesses to allergies and antioxidants – in a comprehensive, easy-to-follow format.

Why should we eat organic food? What are the local varieties, and should we eat them in favour of food that has travelled thousands of miles? How do our needs change as we get older? How much meat should we eat and, if we don't eat it, is it healthy to be a vegetarian?

We are on the brink of a new era, and using this book as your guide to a nutritious, healthy diet and way of life, you can greet it with health and vitality.

The elements of a healthy diet

WHAT IS FOOD?

Food is the fuel for the human body. It is made up of specific elements – proteins, carbohydrates, fats, vitamins, minerals and water – all of which are necessary for life, growth, body function and tissue repair. Traditionally, foods come from animal or plant sources but the rise in food processing has led to an increase in chemically created 'artificial' foods.

Manufacturers have decided that natural food is uninspiring, and have jazzed it up with the addition of a huge number of different ingredients to make it look better. They process things to make them last longer, and to make them easier to eat and prepare. On the whole, convenience is an asset, but what's the cost?

Many highly processed or chemically created foods provide us with energy in the form of calories, which means that we are able to survive by eating them. But they lack vitamins, minerals, fibre and other important elements, which means that in the long run we can become ill from nutritional deficiency.

Following a healthy diet can make you look and feel well, and it ensures that your body is working at optimum level.

A HEALTHY DIET

A healthy diet is one in which the food you eat contains all the nutrients needed by the body for it to grow, heal, and undertake all of the processes necessary to life. Any one food may contain several of these essential nutrients, together with the substances needed to assist their absorption.

These essential nutrients are broken into two main groups: 'macronutrients', which include fats, carbohydrates and protein, and 'micronutrients', which include vitamins, minerals and other trace elements.

• **Macronutrient**s produce energy, and are required in quantities easily measurable by common kitchen scales.

• In contrast, vitamins and minerals are often referred to as the **micronutrients** which, despite their essential nature, are only required in very small, or 'microscopic' amounts. Micronutrients do not produce energy, but they are necessary for the body to release it.

The average Western diet is high in cholesterol and fats, particularly saturated fats, low in fibre, and high in refined sugars and animal products. Diets that are low in fat and cholesterol, and high in dietary fibre, fruits and vegetables produce healthier people, who have much more energy.

Typical Western diet

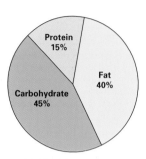

Recommended diet

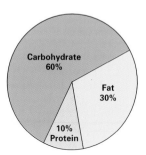

INCREASING THE NUTRIENT VALUE OF YOUR FOOD

The most nutritious foods are fresh foods, with the minimum of processing. As food ages, it becomes less healthy, with fewer 'active' nutrients, especially vitamins and minerals. It is, therefore, important to preserve the nutritional content of your food whenever possible. Keep food fresh:

- Eat brown, unpolished rice and whole grains wherever possible. Refined foods have up to 80 percent fewer nutrients, and much less fibre.

- Choose fresh fruit and vegetables first, but remember that nutritional value decreases with age. Frozen is a better option if you aren't going to eat the food immediately. Fresh foods that have sat on a supermarket shelf, or in the back of a lorry for several days, will be far less nutritious than those from a local market that normally receives daily deliveries fresh from a farm.

- Eat raw whenever possible; if you do cook your fruit and vegetables, use as little water as possible because

---

REMEMBER

To get the most nutrition from your food:

- Brown instead of white
- Fresh or frozen instead of tinned
- Raw instead of cooked vegetables
- With skins instead of peeled

many nutrients are killed by heat or boiled out of food into the water.

- Eat organic food. It may be a little more expensive, but you can be sure that it has been grown without the use of pesticides and other chemicals. Organic food also tastes better!

- Eat the skins of fruits and vegetables (apart from carrots, which can absorb toxins from the soil). Wash them carefully first.

- Don't cut, wash or soak fruits and vegetables until you are ready to eat them. Exposing their cut surfaces to air reduces many nutrients.

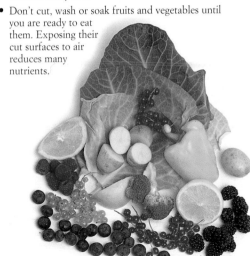

Fats

Fat has become a fairly contentious issue. We know that fat is one of the 'macronutrients', and that we need it for energy. It also has other roles in the body, and some fat is essential for good health. What we need to be concerned with is the *type* of fat we eat, and the *quantity* in which we eat it.

WHAT ARE FATS?

Fats in our food are a prime source of energy and ensure the smooth functioning of the body, in particular the nervous system. They contain the vitamins A and D and are found in meat, fish, dairy produce and vegetable oils.

Fat is stored by our bodies in special cells which tend to form pads of tissue under the skin, and around certain organs and joints, protecting us from shocks and jolts and providing insulation. And one advantage of fat is that it insulates you against the cold and keeps you warm!

A BUILT-IN ENERGY SUPPLY

Stored fat is a concentrated source of energy and it serves as fuel for our bodies. The breakdown of stored fat provides energy for the muscles to contract. A healthy man might have about 33 lb (15 kg) of stored fat, which theoretically can support life for about two months. Obese people may have as much as 220 lb (100 kg) of fat – effectively a year's supply! Research has

HOW MUCH FAT DO YOU NEED?

The general opinion is that we need to eat less of all types of fat, and also change the balance between unsaturated and saturated. Most people in the West take about 40 to 65 percent of their diet as fat and in Britain it is recommended that fat should provide no more than 30 to 35 percent of a diet. In countries such as Sweden and Canada, even lower proportions have been recommended. In line with recent research, the current recommendation is about 30 percent, of which the majority should be unsaturated (mono-unsaturated or polyunsaturated). For tips on how to figure out the percentage of fat in your diet, *see* pp 24-5.

shown that fat distribution in men and women serves different purposes: abdominal fat, found more often in men, provides fuel for quick energy, while the fat in the thighs and buttocks of women provides energy for pregnancy and breastfeeding.

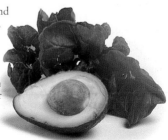

SATURATED AND UNSATURATED FATS

The terms 'saturated' and 'unsaturated' refer to the chemical bonding structure within the fatty acid:

- A saturated fat tends to be more solid than an unsaturated one at room temperature. An example of saturated fat is butter or the fat on the outside of meat. Saturated fats usually come from an animal source (coconut oil is the exception to this rule).

- An unsaturated fat tends to be more liquid at room temperature. Unsaturated fats usually come from plant sources and include corn oil and sunflower oil.

Unsaturated fats are broken down into two further groups: *poly*unsaturated and *mono*unsaturated. **Monounsaturates** include things like olive oil and avocados, and **polyunsaturates** are found in corn, sunflower seeds, peanuts and other foods, from which they are extracted.

BAD FATS

A high intake of saturated fats – animal fats – has been linked to many diseases, including heart disease, stroke, obesity and cancer. Saturated fat clogs the arteries and interferes with the body's metabolism, adding extra weight and preventing the absorption of beneficial nutrients

Unsaturated fat, while better for you than saturated fat, is not without its risks. Polyunsaturated vegetable margarines and shortenings, and 'half-fat' spreads are usually **hydrogenated**, which means that they are processed to change them from liquids (oils) to solid or semi-solid fats. What should be healthy fats become artificially produced saturated fats, with most of the same problems associated with animal fats. Consumption of hydrogenated fat has been linked to cancer, heart disease and other conditions.

Read the label when you shop. If it says 'hydrogenated vegetable oil', don't buy it.

WHAT TO DO:

Use:

- Olive oil instead of lard
- Pure vegetable oil margarine instead of hydrogenated ones
- Stir-fry instead of deep-frying
- Keep animal fats – meat and dairy produce – to a minimum

Good fats

Good fats are normally 'polyunsaturated' or 'monounsaturated': those found in olive oil, for example, are monounsaturated; polyunsaturated fats include those found in fish, nuts, and seeds. Monounsaturates appear to have a protective function against heart disease. This concept partly explains the 'French' or 'Mediterranean' paradox, where nations of smokers and drinkers, eating a diet that is often high in fat, suffer from comparatively little heart disease. The healthy oils, such as olive oil, seem to prevent heart disease, and to lower cholesterol in the body that could lead to cardiovascular problems.

Essential fatty acids

Certain polyunsaturates are 'essential'. This means that the body cannot make them from other dietary fats or oils and, therefore, we must get them from our food. The two main essential polyunsaturates are **linoleic acid** and **linolenic acid**.

These oils are found naturally in fresh foods, such as seeds, nuts, vegetables and fish, and even in wild meat such as game. For optimum health, you need 2–4 tablespoons of these essential fatty acids every day, but despite our high consumption of fat, they can be hard to find in the Western diet.

Seeds, especially sesame and sunflower seeds, are rich in **linoleic acid** (also known as Omega-6), while pumpkin and flax seeds are rich in **linoleic acid** (Omega-3). Whilst many people could benefit from a diet lower in fat, we must all eat some fat to maintain health. A completely fat-free diet is potentially dangerous. In fact, several recent studies have shown that some very fit athletes, for whom fats comprise less than 15 percent of daily calorie intake (instead of 30 percent), suffer from problems with their immune systems.

Make sure you include some of the 'good fats' listed below in your diet every day.

WHAT ARE THE GOOD FATS?

Good fats contain essential fatty acids.

Choose from:

- olive oil (monounsaturated fatty acid)
- sesame seeds, and sunflower seeds (Omega-6)
- pumpkin and linseeds (Omega-3)
- fish oils
- evening primrose and borage

CUTTING DOWN ON FAT

The best way to avoid fatty foods is to read the labels. All labels (*see* pp 144-8) should give you an idea of the fat content per serving, although some labels show this as a proportion of the whole package. You'll also need to get to know which foods are fatty, and which aren't, and try to ensure that the healthy fats (the unsaturates) are much more prominent in your diet than the unhealthy fats (the saturates).

High-fat foods	Low-fat alternatives
Butter	Vegetable margarine
Whole milk	Skimmed milk
Cheddar cheese	Feta or cottage cheese
Cream cheese dips	Low-fat yoghurt dips
Mayonnaise	Salad dressing of lemon juice or balsamic vinegar
Peanut butter	Jams or jellies
Fried foods	Baked or steamed foods
Fatty, 'marbled' meats	Trimmed, lean meats
Chicken with skin	Chicken without skin
Creamy sauces	Mustard, chutneys, marinades
Crisps	Air-popped popcorn
Doughnuts	Rice cakes

The following list shows how easily it is possible for you to reduce your fat intake just by switching to a lower-fat product:

Food	Cals.	Fat (g)	Sat. fat (g)
Light tuna, in oil (100g/4oz)	226	9	2
Light tuna, in brine (100g/4oz)	150	2	0
Whole milk (250ml/8oz)	150	8	5
Semi-skimmed milk (250ml/8oz)	120	5	4
Skimmed milk (250ml/8oz)	80	trace	trace
Cheddar cheese (30g/1oz)	115	9	6
Feta cheese (30g/1oz)	75	6	4
Cottage cheese (30g/1oz)	108	5	3
Low-fat cottage cheese (30g/1oz)	104	2	1
Plain whole milk yoghurt (30g/1oz)	139	7	5
Plain low-fat yoghurt (30g/1oz)	143	4	2
Butter (individual pat; 10g/½oz)	74	8.2	4.7
Margarine, soft (individual pat: 10g/½oz)	73	8.1	2.5

Here's an example of a high-fat daily menu:

Food	Cal.	Fat (g)
BREAKFAST		
Bacon, grilled, 2 rashers	292	18.9
Sausage, fried, 2 large	254	19.7
Eggs, fried in butter, 2	184	14.5
Croissant with 1 pat butter	333	24
Coffee with cream	20	2
MIDMORNING SNACK		
Milk chocolate, 50g	265	15.2
LUNCH		
Burger, quarter pounder	413	20.7
Chips, 150g	378	16.4
AFTERNOON SNACK		
Doughnut	262	11.9
Coffee with cream	20	2
DINNER		
Roast beef, brisket, 100g	367	30
Roast potatoes, 2 medium	173	5.3
Yorkshire pudding	225	12.5
Peas, tinned, 1 serving	47	0.3
Sponge cake, 50g	23	13.3
Custard, 2 tbsp	47	2.4

The **total calories** for the day: 3512
Total fat grams: 209.1 (the maximum recommended is 80g)

Fat percentage = 209.1 ÷ 3512 x 100% = 59.5%

Here's an example of a menu with 30% fat content:

Food	Cal.	Fat (g)
BREAKFAST		
Oatmeal (90g cooked)	145	2.5
Banana	104	0.5
Wholemeal toast		
with 1 tbsp butter	161	11
MIDMORNING SNACK		
½ cinnamon and raisin bagel		
with 25g cream cheese	256	10
LUNCH		
Tuna sandwich with mayonnaise		
on wholewheat bread)	404	16
Low-fat baked tortilla chips (25g)	110	1
AFTERNOON SNACK		
6 ginger snaps	180	4
DINNER		
Prawn kebabs (250g): prawns,		
red or green peppers, onions,		
barbecue sauce or marinade	301	4
Steamed brown rice (75g)	108	1
Steamed broccoli and carrots		
with 2 tbsp parmesan cheese	112	4
Sponge cake with 75g strawberries	139	6

Therefore, the **total calories** for the day: 2020
Total fat grams: 60
Fat percentage = 60 ÷ 2020 x 100% = 30 percent

EAT MORE, WEIGH LESS

Gram for gram, fat has twice the calories of the other two main nutrients – protein and carbohydrate. If you want to lose weight, cut your fat intake down to 20 percent. You will be able to eat more food, while consuming fewer calories.

Look at the daily menu on p. 25 and see where the big fat contributors are. In this case, the cream cheese and the mayonnaise in the tuna sandwich have the highest fat content. If you cut the cream cheese, you have reduced your fat count by about 10 grams. You could eat five bagels, which are naturally low in fat, and still be within your fat total. If you cut the mayonnaise from your tuna fish, and added dill and fat-free mayonnaise instead, you could, theoretically, eat almost seven tuna sandwiches for the same amount of fat.

FAT-FREE ALTERNATIVES

Many of the fat-free or fat-reduced alternatives contain a host of extra ingredients, some of which are not very healthy. However, if you are eating a good, balanced diet, with plenty of fresh, whole foods, fat-free treats are perfectly acceptable. In balance, it is better to keep the fat content of your diet low, preventing heart disease, obesity and other health problems.

CHOLESTEROL

More has been written about the good and bad effects of cholesterol over the past ten years than almost any other health issue. Here are the facts:

WHAT IS CHOLESTEROL?

Cholesterol is a white, waxy, fatlike substance that occurs in our body tissues. Excess cholesterol can build up in the bloodstream and accumulate on the walls of arteries, forming 'plaques' which can clog the blood vessels and lead to heart attacks and stroke. There is much debate as to correct levels of cholesterol in the blood and how to reduce cholesterol in the diet.

Cholesterol is important for several reasons. It is stored in the adrenal glands, testes, and ovaries, and converted to steroid hormones. Cholesterol helps the liver make bile, which is necessary to digest food, especially fats. It

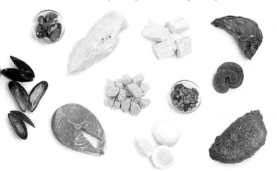

also insulates our nerves and has many other functions in the body. We need cholesterol. The problem is, we get too much of it.

WE MAKE OUR OWN CHOLESTEROL!

All animals, including humans, make their own cholesterol. In fact, we make all the cholesterol that we need. Where trouble sets in is when we take in too much *extra* cholesterol in our diets.

Cholesterol is found in animal products – in other words, foods that contain saturated fats. If we eat too much of them, our cholesterol levels are increased and we are at risk of heart disease and other problems.

MEASURING CHOLESTEROL

When you have your cholesterol levels checked, either at the doctor, or in the chemist, you are looking for the number of milligrams of cholesterol per decilitre of blood. Most experts suggest that cholesterol levels for people under 30 should be less than 150 mg/dl. Over 30, 180 mg/dl. If your cholesterol is too high, consult your doctor about methods of reducing it.

Carbohydrates

Carbohydrates, which include cellulose, starches, sugars, and many other compounds, are the greatest dietary source of energy. Important dietary carbohydrates are divided into two groups – starches and sugars.

The starches, which are converted into sugars in the body, are found in grains, pulses, tubers (such as potatoes), and some roots (carrots, for example). The sugars occur in many plants and fruits, the most important being sucrose, which is obtained from sugar cane or the sugar beet.

SUGARS

The most common simple sugars are glucose, fructose and galactose. The major sources of sugar in the diet are sugar added to food and drink, soft drinks and sweets. Sugar is also added to a wide range of processed foods, including soups, tinned fruits and vegetables, baked

---

THE HEALTHY EATING CARBOHYDRATE SCALE

Excellent fruit, vegetables, wholegrains (brown rice, wholemeal bread), pulses (lentils, beans, barley etc.)

Fair white rice, white flour, white bread, pasta

Poor sugar, honey, icecream, chocolate, fizzy drinks, puddings

beans and some meat products, although these sources do not add much to the diet. In the UK between 14 and 26 percent of most people's diet is sugar.

Sugars provide calories and no other nutrients. If you fill up on sugary foods, you are likely to be at risk of tooth decay, and vitamin and mineral deficiencies.

STARCHES

Starches, which are also known as 'complex carbohydrates', are found principally in plant foods. Starch is the plant's energy store and fibre is the packaging of the plant cell wall that makes it tough and

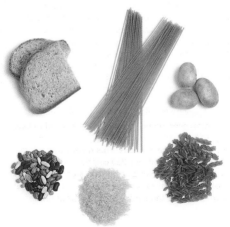

gives it its shape. Highly refined starches, like cornflour or white flour, have as little nutritional value as sugars. However, unrefined starches, such as wholegrain bread, wholegrain or brown flours, pasta, beans and potatoes are also a good source of protein and a wide range of vitamins and minerals. Whole, or unrefined, foods are also a very good source of fibre (*see* p. 34).

SUGARS VERSUS STARCHES

Any carbohydrates will give the body energy. However, the types of carbohydrate you eat can have an effect on your mood and your energy level.

Sugar carbohydrates tend to give us a sudden burst of energy, followed by a slump, whereas starches, the complex carbohydrates from vegetables, pulses (legumes), seeds, and fruit, provide more sustained energy over a longer period of time. The slow-release mechanism in complex carbohydrates works to prevent drastic swings in blood sugar level.

HOW MUCH SUGAR DO YOU NEED?

Experts recommend that sugar be reduced to less than 10 percent of your total daily calorie intake, and not eaten between meals. This means that adults should not exceed 150–250 calories a day from sugar. If you eat two biscuits, a pot of sweetened yoghurt and have four cups of tea with a spoonful of sugar in each, then you've reached your limit.

INCREASING YOUR CONSUMPTION OF STARCHES

Many countries with a lower incidence of heart disease
and bowel cancer than the UK and the US have a much
higher intake of complex carbohydrates. Most of us
plan our meals by choosing the meat, or equivalent,
first. We need to rethink how we eat, by building upon
a base of starchy staples, such as jacket potatoes, brown
rice or wholemeal pasta.

Here are some tips for increasing the level of complex
carbohydrates in your diet:

- Plan meals by selecting the carbohydrate (such as rice,
  couscous or potatoes) first. Then choose vegetables,
  and finally the meat or fish.

HOW MUCH STARCH DO YOU NEED?

In the West, the starch carbohydrates we eat
normally take the form of pasta, bread, flour and
potatoes, and carbohydrates make up about 45
percent of our diet. Of this, almost half comes from
sugar and the rest from complex carbohydrates.
Experts recommend that we should aim to get at
least 60 percent of our daily calorie intake from
complex carbohydrates, preferably unrefined.

Vegetables, pulses, seeds and fruit should be the
predominant source, with around 10–15 percent of
our calories coming from wholegrains, potatoes,
wholewheat bread and pasta.

- Try to serve wholegrain bread with your meals – without butter or margarine. Fresh, warm bread (why not choose partly baked baguettes from the supermarket?) is delicious on its own, and a great source of complex carbohydrates and fibre (*see* p. 34).

- Eat plenty of potatoes, especially baked in their skin or roasted with the minimum of fat. If chips are your downfall, *see* the box on p. 68.

- Make sure that you eat plenty of bread, particularly wholegrain. Don't give up white pasta, bread, rice or cereals if you don't like the wholegrain alternatives. The emphasis should be on increasing carbohydrates in your diet and these foods do contain them.

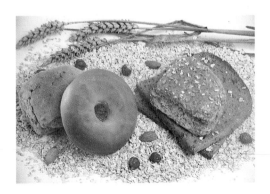

FIBRE

Dietary fibre, also known as bulk and roughage, is an essential part of the diet even though it provides no nutrients. It consists of plant cellulose and other indigestible materials in foods, along with pectin and gum.

Fruits, vegetables, wholegrain breads, and products made from nuts and pulses are all sources of dietary fibre. In fact, practically all foods of plant origin are useful sources of dietary fibre. (Sugar is an exception as it is a highly purified extract from cane and beet.) White bread usually has only about 3 percent fibre. The richest sources of fibre are wholemeal bread and flour, peas, beans, dried fruits and nuts.

What does fibre do?

The chewing fibre requires stimulates saliva flow, and the bulk it adds in the stomach and intestines during digestion aids absorption of nutrients. Diets with sufficient fibre produce softer, bulkier stools and help to promote bowel regularity. There is also some evidence that a fibre-rich diet can prevent cancers of the bowel and other parts of the digestive tract.

Pectin, which is a soluble fibre found in apples and carrots, is particularly useful for absorbing heavy metals, such as lead, and preventing them from being absorbed. It also encourages efficient elimination of waste products, and prevents the reabsorption of toxins in the bowel. Pectin also helps to balance blood sugar levels.

Fibre is particularly important in the control of the body's cholesterol levels. If your diet includes sufficient natural fibre, any excess cholesterol will be excreted along with all the other waste materials. That's good news, if your diet tends to contain foods with lots of

FIBRE-RICH FOODS

apples	green beans
aubergines	linseeds (flax seed)
bananas	muesli
beets	oatmeal
bran	peas
bran (rice)	peppers
broccoli	potatoes
Brussels sprouts	radishes
cabbage	sesame seeds
carrots	squash
cauliflower	strawberries
citrus fruit (pith)	wholegrain flour
grapes	

cholesterol.

A HIGH-FIBRE DIET

A 'high-fibre' diet does not mean adding bran to every meal. In fact, bran is harsh on the digestive tract and can result in many important minerals being excreted from the body along with waste materials. The fibre in vegetables, fruit, oats, lentils and beans is much more gentle and effective.

Increasing fibre intake

• Make sure that your diet includes a variety of fibre-rich foods, such as green and salad vegetables, root vegetables, fresh fruit, cereals, nuts, pulses and wholegrain foods.

• Include some raw fruit and vegetables, which have the

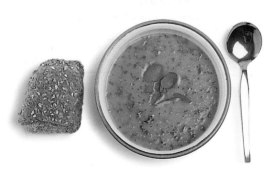

HOW MUCH FIBRE DO YOU NEED?

Most experts recommend that we get 25 to 30 grams (1 oz) of fibre every day. The precise amount will vary in proportion to the number of calories you take. This might be equivalent to a bowl of bran cereal, a baked potato, an apple, 3 slices of wholemeal bread, a portion each of broccoli and carrots, a banana and a portion of brown rice. Try to eat at least 10 portions of fibre-rich foods a day and you should be getting enough.

highest fibre content.

- Choose wholegrain products such as brown rice, wholemeal pasta, wholemeal bread and rolls and wholemeal breakfast cereals.

- Sprinkle sesame seeds on salads and add dried fruits to breakfast cereals.

- Include more beans and pulses in your diet. In many meals you can replace the meat with beans or lentils.

- Eat potatoes baked in their jackets. The jackets are not only high in fibre, but they contain lots of vitamin C.

Proteins

Protein provides the nutrients for maintaining the structure of your body. About 17 percent of the body is made of protein, including muscles, bones, skin, nails and hair. Protein is made up of differing combinations of 23 separate amino acids, all of which are necessary for life and healthy body functioning.

The human body can produce most of the amino acids it needs, but there are 8 (9 in the case of babies) that it cannot make itself. These are known as the essential amino acids and they must be obtained from proteins in the diet.

THE PROTEIN BALANCE

Generally, a lack of protein in the diet retards growth in children and causes a decrease in energy. Excess protein intake on the other hand puts a strain on the liver and kidneys, and leads to an increased risk of certain cancers and coronary heart disease.

GETTING ENOUGH PROTEIN

Most people in the West get enough protein. In fact, one study showed that Americans eat between twice and eight times as much as they need! However, with recent research showing how harmful fats can be, we are now advised to get as much protein as we can from non-animal sources. That means increasing our of intake of vegetable proteins, which is easier than you'd think.

Virtually all unrefined foods are loaded with proteins. For example, rice is 8 percent protein, oranges are 8 percent, potatoes are 10 percent and beans are 26 percent. Wheat comes in at 16 percent, as does oatmeal.

Animal proteins	Vegetable proteins
Beef, pork, lamb	Quorn and other meat substitutes
Bacon, ham, sausages	Tofu
Chicken, turkey, game	Pasta
Fish and seafood	Stringbeans
Milk, butter, cheese	Broccoli
Eggs	Seedless raisins
	Sweetcorn
	Black beans
	Pulses
	Brown rice
	Sweet cherries
	Bananas

HOW MUCH PROTEIN DO YOU NEED?

It is recommended that about 15 percent of the daily calorie intake should come from proteins. The average adult doesn't need more than 2 oz (60 g) of protein per day. This is equivalent to a piece of meat or chicken less than the size of this book!

Take a look at the menu ideas for vegetarians on p. 124. If you can swap one or two meat courses a week for vegetarian options, you'll be well on your way to ensuring that you are getting the right kind of proteins in your diet.

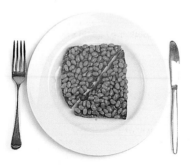

A NOTE ABOUT SALT

We eat approximately 10 grams of salt every day, and ideally should reduce this to about 5 grams. There is some evidence that too much salt can cause high blood pressure, although this is by no means certain. We do know that some people are sensitive to excessive salt, and they are more likely to suffer from water retention (oedema) and heart problems.

Most of the salt we eat has been added to foods, either by the manufacturer, or from table salt. Eliminating table salt entirely will knock about 5 grams off your daily intake. Eliminating foods that contain added salt, such as crisps, will get you close to the desired goal. Many products are now available that are only lightly salted, and people are getting used to cooking with herbs and spices, which have no salt, but which still add taste and variety to your food.

The following foods are high in salt:
crisps
cheese
bacon
ham
tinned and packet soups
yeast extracts
soda water
smoked meat and fish
salted peanuts
tinned fish

Vitamins and minerals

Vitamins are compounds needed by the body in small quantities to enable it to grow, develop and function. They work with other compounds, to help produce energy, build tissues, remove waste, and ensure that each system works efficiently.

Minerals are metals and other inorganic compounds, which work in much the same way as vitamins, promoting body processes, and providing much of the structure for teeth and bones. Minerals are classified in two groups – proper, or major minerals, needed in quantities of over 100mg per day, and minor minerals, or trace elements, which are required by the body in quantities less than 100mg per day.

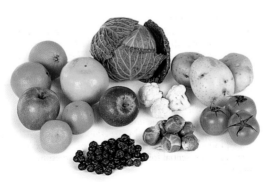

WHAT ARE RDAS?

RDA stands for the Recommended Daily Dietary Allowance, established by government health organisations. RDAs are the levels of nutrients believed to be adequate to meet the needs of a healthy individual. They are not the levels necessary for **optimum** health, as they are based on the needs of the average healthy person.

Different countries recommend different levels, but the RDAs shown in our Vitamin and Minerals charts on pp 46-52 are those recommended by the EU.

Vitamins and minerals work together and require the actions of other vitamins and minerals to be effective.

TYPES OF VITAMINS

The vitamins needed by humans are divided into water-soluble vitamins (B vitamins and vitamin C) and fat-soluble vitamins (A, D, E, and K). When you take in more water-soluble vitamins than are needed most of the excess is excreted in your urine so you need to include them in your daily diet to prevent depletion.

Fat-soluble vitamins have highly specialized functions: they are absorbed by the intestine, and carried to the different parts of the body by the lymphatic system, which forms part of your immune system. Fat-soluble vitamins are essential for maintaining the structure of our cells.

GETTING ENOUGH

A diet that has enough fresh, unrefined foods should have adequate quantities of vitamins and minerals. Fresh fruits, vegetables and salads should appear in your daily diet, and fresh meat and fish should be used in the place of packaged or frozen foods.

Many of the processes used to preserve good, such as freezing and canning, can result in a loss of nutrients. Wherever possible, try to choose goods that are fresh and local, since long storage or periods of travelling, can cause nutrients to be lost. Many product labels list the vitamin and mineral content of food.

If you eat a diet that isn't as fresh or wholesome as it should be, look out for foods with extra vitamins and minerals added. This simply means that nutrients lost in the processing have been added back – usually not in the same quantities, but it will help ensure that you get what you need.

SUPPLEMENTING VITAMINS AND MINERALS

Some experts now believe that supplementing our diet with vitamin and mineral tablets is sensible. It is estimated that more than 50 percent of the population of the USA and the UK take supplements. Most people will benefit from a good multi-vitamin or mineral supplement, which will help ensure that any imbalances in your diet are righted before they cause health problems.

VITAMINS

A

Sources: Organ meats (liver and kidney), eggs, butter, fish oils; and betacarotene found in dark green and yellow fruits and vegetables. **Function:** Needed for strong bones, good vision and healthy skin; improves the body's ability to heal. An antioxidant (*see* p. 49).

RDA: 700mcg (2300iu)

Caution: May cause birth defects if taken during pregnancy.

B1 (THIAMINE)

Sources: All plant and animal foods, including wholegrain products, brown rice, seafood and beans. **Function:** Converts blood sugar into energy, promotes growth and is a nerve tonic.

RDA: 1mg

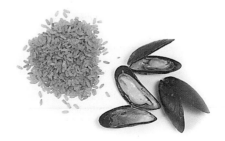

B2 (RIBOFLAVIN)

Sources: Milk and dairy produce, green leafy vegetables, liver, kidneys and yeast. **Function:** An antioxidant (*see* p. 49). Aids in cell respiration, growth and reproduction. Essential for the body to produce energy. **RDA:** 1.3mg

B3 (NIACIN)

Sources: Meats, fish and poultry, wholegrains, peanuts and avocados. **Function:** Essential for sex hormones, increases energy, aids nervous system, helps digestion. **RDA:** 18mg

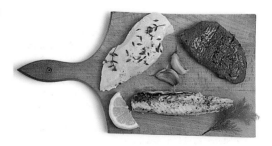

B5 (PANTOTHENIC ACID)

Sources: Organ meats, fish, eggs, chicken, nuts and wholegrain cereals. **Function:** Aids in healing wounds, fights infection, strengthens immune system, builds cells. **RDA:** 7mg (estimated adequate intake)

B6 (Pyridoxine, Pyridoxal-5-Phosphate)

Sources: Meats, eggs, wholegrains, yeast, cabbage, melon and molasses.

Function: Required for the functioning of more than 60 enzymes, aids the nervous system and the production of cells. Crucial for a healthy immune system and for the production of antibodies and white blood cells.

RDA: 1.5mg

B12 (Cyanocolbalamin)

Sources: Fish, dairy produce, beef, pork, lamb, organ

MEGADOSING

Many health practitioners believe that some vitamins can be taken in excess for their therapeutic qualities, or in large 'megadoses'. In general, it is not wise to supplement too much of one vitamin, for it throws out the balance of the others. Vitamins interact with each other in the body to fulfil their various roles. Too much of one can deplete another, or make its action ineffective. If you wish to megadose, only do so under the supervision of a registered health professional.

There are some exceptions to this rule. In the case of a cold or viral infection, for instance, extra Vitamin C can substantially reduce the duration of the illness. It is water-soluble, so any excess will be excreted in the urine.

meats, eggs and milk. **Function:** Forms red
blood cells, increases energy, improves memory and
concentration, maintains nervous system, promotes
healthy growth in children. **RDA:** 1.5mcg

FOLIC ACID (VITAMIN Bc)

Sources: Fresh leafy green vegetables, yeasts and liver,
carrots, avocado and apricots. **Function:** Essential for
red blood cells, metabolism of sugar, protects against
fetal abnormalities; amino acids and manufacture of
antibodies, crucial to the nervous system and for the
production of DNA and RNA. **RDA:** 200mcg

C (ASCORBIC ACID)

Sources: Fresh fruit and vegetables, potatoes, leafy
herbs and berries. **Function:** Vital for healthy skin,
bones, muscles, healing and protection from viruses and
allergies, good vision. Necessary for cholesterol metabolism. An effective antioxidant (*see* p. 49). **RDA:** 40mg

D

Sources: Milk produce,
eggs, fatty fish, fish oil.
Synthesized in the skin
from sunlight.
Function: Vital for
growth, and health
of bones and teeth.
Increases absorption of
calcium from diet.
RDA: none

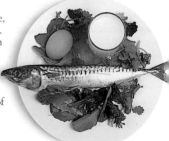

E

Sources: Nuts, seeds, eggs, milk, wholegrains, unrefined oils, leafy vegetables, avocados, and soya. **Function:** Necessary for absorption of iron, metabolism of essential fatty acids, protects the circulatory system and cells, slows ageing, increases fertility and protects

---

ANTIOXIDANTS

Nutrients called antioxidants – vitamins C, E and beta-carotene, and the minerals Zinc and Selenium, among others – are now known to have an anti-ageing effect. Contained in fruits, nuts and most vegetables, antioxidants are the body's defence against what scientists call 'free radicals'.

In small quantities free radicals can fight bacteria and viruses; in larger quantities they encourage the ageing process and cause damage to our cells. Free radicals are implicated in the initiation of cancer and heart disease. Many experts believe that the ageing process is actually produced by the constant, tiny degenerative effects caused by free radicals as they oxidize various cells over time.

Both vitamin E and vitamin C are powerful antioxidants, and are highly efficient at mopping up free radicals. Recently, it has been discovered that vitamin A, Selenium, Zinc and Copper are also effective antioxidants.

against fetal abnormalities. An antioxidant (*see* p. 47).
RDA: none at present

K
Sources: Green vegetables, milk products, molasses, apricots, whole grains, cod liver oil. Synthezised in the intestines. **Function:** Produces blood-clotting factors.
RDA: none

MAJOR MINERALS

CALCIUM

Sources: Dairy produce, leafy green vegetables, salmon, nuts, root vegetables, broccoli and tofu. **Function:** Necessary for hormones and muscles, aids nervous system. Necessary for blood clotting and blood pressure regulation; maintains strong bones and teeth. Helps to metabolize iron. **RDA:** 700mg

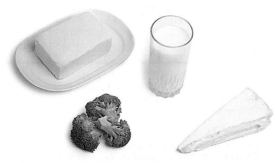

CHROMIUM

Sources: Liver, wholegrain cereals, meat and cheese, brewer's yeast, molasses, mushrooms and egg yolk.
Function: Stimulates insulin activity. **RDA:** 25mcg (minimum suggested intake)

IODINE

Sources: Fish and seafood, pineapple, raisins, seaweed, dairy produce. **Function:** Produces hormones from the thyroid gland. Promotes healthy hair, skin, nails and teeth. **RDA:** 140mcg

IRON

Sources: Liver, kidney, raw clams, cocoa powder, dark chocolate, shellfish, pulses, broccoli and dark green vegetables, nuts, egg yolks, red meat, beans and molasses. **Function:** Necessary for production of haemoglobin and certain enzymes. Necessary for immune activity and to supply oxygen to the cells.
RDA: 14.8mg (women); 8.7mg (men)

MAGNESIUM

Sources: brown rice, soya beans, nuts, brewer's yeast, whole grains, bitter chocolate and legumes. **Function:** Repairs and maintains body cells. Required for most body processes, and transmission of nerve impulses; growth and repair and bone development.
RDA: 300mg.

POTASSIUM

Sources: Avocados, leafy green vegetables, bananas, dried fruits, fruit and vegetable juices, soya flour, potatoes, nuts and molasses. **Function:** Necessary for transportation of carbon dioxide by red blood cells. Required for water balance and protein synthesis, nerve and muscle function. **RDA:** 3500mg.

These are the primiary minerals to include in your diet. If you are getting enough of them, your other mineral needs will almost certainly be met as well. Some mineral waters are good sources of minerals (*see* pp 162-3).

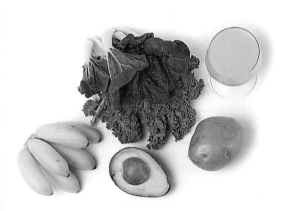

Example of a daily menu that supplies necessary vitamins and minerals:

BREAKFAST
Glass of fresh orange juice; 1 poached egg on wholemeal toast; muesli with sultanas, roasted seeds and nuts; sliced banana

SNACK
1 peach; 2 oat flapjacks with sultanas; tea with lemon

LUNCH
Roasted vegetables with low-fat mozzarella on a wholegrain bap; mug of potato and leek soup (optional)
1 carton low-fat fruit yoghurt; banana; apple juice

SNACK
1 apple; half wholemeal muffin with peanut butter; peppermint tea

DINNER
Grilled chicken with lemon and thyme; brown rice with a handful of wild rice added; salad of lettuce, tomatoes, cucumber, red peppers, avocado and black olives with low-fat French dressing, sprinkled with ½ a handful of toasted sesame seeds; sweetcorn
6 chocolate-covered brazil nuts; fruit salad with mango, apple, clementine and grapes in a little apple juice; spring water, or a glass of red wine

Planning balanced meals

The most important aspect of healthy eating is balance. Eating all the right foods and denying yourself the occasional treat is bound to make you long for things on the 'taboo' list and make it less likely that you'll be able to maintain a healthy eating regime.

Eating should be a pleasure. Enjoy your food, and take time to prepare it. Choose luscious green salads with chunks of marinated chicken, raw sugar-snap peas, fresh red onion, peppers, and grated carrot. Top it off with a delicious French dressing. Add some crusty wholegrain bread, and you have a perfectly balanced meal. If you concentrate on the fruits and vegetables, and then the carbohydrate and protein parts of your meals, you'll find that most meals you prepare are naturally lower in fat and filling.

It is how you combine foods together each day and each week that is important. All foods can be enjoyed as part of a healthy eating plan if they are eaten in reasonable amounts.

THE FOOD PYRAMID

Over the years, research into nutrition has led to the concept of a food pyramid, which shows daily diet recommendations in the form of a diagram. Foods that should be eaten more often are at the base, and those used less frequently at the top. The emphasis is on consuming less meat and meat substitutes, dairy products and oils and fats, and more breads and cereals, and fruits and vegetables. Some scientists feel that these recommendations do not go far enough and are pressing for the near elimination of meats and fats from the Western diet.

UNDERSTANDING THE FOOD PYRAMID

The Food Guide Pyramid is a practical tool to help you make food choices that are consistent with the dietary guidelines recommended by the government. Using the pyramid enables you to eat a variety of foods daily so that you can get the nutrients you need.

Others,
including
sweets, biscuits,
fast foods and cakes
(rarely)

Meat, fish and alternatives
(not more than twice daily)

Milk, cheese and yoghurt
(not more than 3 times daily)

Fruits and vegetables (5–9 times daily)

Bread, cereals and potatoes (6+ times daily)

To make the most of the Pyramid, you need to know what counts as a serving.

Food group	Serving size
Bread	1 slice bread, ½ bagel or muffin, 25g/1oz ready-to-eat cereal, ½ cup porridge, rice or pasta, or 5–6 crackers or oatcakes
Vegetable	1 cup raw, leafy vegetables, ½ cup cooked or chopped raw vegetables or 180ml/6oz vegetable juice
Fruit	1 medium piece of fruit, ½ cup mixed fruit or 180ml/6oz fruit juice
Milk	180ml/6oz milk or yogurt, 40g/1½ oz natural cheese or 60g/2oz processed cheese
Meat	50–75g/2–3oz cooked lean meat, poultry or fish (about the size of a deck of playing cards)

Other foods that count as a serving from the second top row include: ½ cup cooked dry beans, 1 egg, 2 tablespoons of peanut butter or ⅓ cup nuts.

To measure a cup of any food, use a standard-sized coffee or tea mug and fill to the top, but not overflowing.

Here's an example of a daily menu that balances the food groups according to the **Food Pyramid**:

BREAKFAST
Bowl of sultana bran (carbohydrate and fruit)
Sliced banana (fruit)
Milk on cereal (dairy)
2 slices wholegrain toast (carbohydrate x 2)
1 glass fresh apple juice (fruit)

SNACK
Apple (fruit)
Cinnamon and raisin bagel (carbohydrate and fruit)
Scraping of low-fat soft cheese (dairy)

LUNCH
Wholegrain sandwich with tuna, light mayonnaise with sweetcorn, cucumber and salad (2 x carbohydrate, fish, 2 x vegetables)
2 plums (2 x fruit)
Glass fresh orange juice (2 x fruit)

SNACK
Cup of chamomile tea with honey (1 top serving)
2 oat flapjacks (carbohydrate)

DINNER
2 baked potatoes (carbohydrate x 2)
Grilled chicken breasts (meat)
Green salad (vegetables)
Carrots and green beans (2 x vegetables)
Fruit salad (fruit)

TEN TIPS FOR HEALTHY EATING

The following guidelines will help you to shop for food and plan your meals in advance.

1 **Eat a variety of different foods using the food pyramid as a guide** No one food contains all the vitamins, minerals, fibre, protein and energy you need for good health, so you have to eat a range of foods to get the right amount. Use the **Food Pyramid** (*see* p.55) as a guide when making your shopping list.

2 **Eat the right amount of food to be a healthy weight and exercise regularly** (Bear in mind that the correct weight for any individual will depend on sex, height, and age, among other factors.) Choose foods that provide lots of nourishment, but are low in fat.

3 **Eat at least 5 portions of fruit and vegetables a day.** Fruit and vegetables are high in fibre and packed with vitamins (especially A, C, and E), and minerals. They are also low in calories and virtually fat-free.

4 **Eat more complex carbohydrate foods, including bread, cereals, potatoes, pasta and rice.**

Starchy foods are low in fat, provide many essential vitamins and minerals and are filling.

5 Eat more foods rich in fibre – bread and cereals (especially wholegrain), potatoes, fruit and vegetables.

6 Eat less fats, especially saturated fats. Keep a close eye on the amount and type of fat there is in the foods you buy. Reading food labels will help you choose brands that are lower in fat.

7 If you drink or eat snacks containing sugar, limit the number of times you have them throughout the day Sugary snacks and drinks taken frequently throughout the day are a major contributing factor to tooth decay.

8 Use a variety of seasonings

9 Drink alcohol sensibly and preferably with meals Alcohol has become a part of our culture, and studies have shown that a daily drink can enhance rather than destroy your health (*see* p. 166).

10 Enjoy your food and make changes gradually If your favourite foods are high in fat, salt or sugar, the key is to moderate how much you eat of them, without eliminating them altogether. Balance your choices so that over several days they fit together into a healthy pattern. Don't expect to totally revamp your habits overnight. Begin with modest changes that add up over time to a positive, lifelong eating regime.

WHAT IS A BALANCED MEAL?

Using the Food Pyramid as your guide (*see* p. 55), base your meals around the four main categories, ensuring that you have at least 2–3 fruits or vegetables per meal, a little dairy produce (or an alternative, such as soya) and some meat and fish for protein. Make carbohydrates the central feature of your meal. Choose a baked potato with fresh toppings, or chunks of wholemeal bread with fresh vegetables and an olive-oil mayonnaise. Pasta can serve as a main course or a side dish, and adds valuable carbohydrates to your meal.

ADDING VARIETY

The key to balance is variety. Try to choose different fruits and vegetables for each meal. Focus on colour and freshness and you can be assured that they are high in the vitamins and minerals necessary to keep you healthy.

- Don't always eat potatoes with your meal – try couscous, bulgar wheat, wild rice or fresh pasta.

- Eat plenty of fresh fish or lean chicken, keeping fatty meats to a minimum.

- Choose interesting cheeses – feta is low in fat, as is cottage cheese, and they make good toppings for salads and main courses.

- Allow yourself a treat at the end of your main meal to satisfy any cravings.

PLANNING BALANCED MEALS

Often the hardest part of cooking a meal is deciding what to make. Why not write down the ten favourite meals your family enjoys and rotate them? They probably won't take long to prepare if you know them by heart. (*See* **Evening meal suggestions**, p. 67.) The same applies to packed lunches. Write down your five favourite sandwich fillers or snacks (*see also* **Lunch suggestions** on p. 66).

The principles of a healthy meal or snack have been outlined earlier but in addition to the nutritional aspect of the meal, aesthetic qualities should be considered. Colour, texture and flavour all help to make food enjoyable.

The following suggestions will help you to plan meals that are interesting, tasty, nutritious and easy to prepare.

BREAKFAST

Breakfast has often been described as the most important meal of the day, but there is some debate about that theory. Some research has shown that missing breakfast leads to loss of concentration and impaired performance during the morning. And a recent study showed that children who ate breakfast, especially when cereals were included, managed to have the most nutritious diet. But other studies say that missing breakfast occasionally is more of a problem than going without it regularly. They say that the ill-effects occur when normal routines are disrupted.

No breakfast?

If you don't eat breakfast, try not to eat snacks that are high in fat and sugar and low in fibre, such as chocolate or crisps. People who are dieting often make the mistake of not having breakfast in an attempt to cut down on calories, and they wonder why they are hungry mid-morning! It makes more sense to start the day with a high-fibre and low-fat breakfast than to end up eating an unhealthy snack later. If you don't feel like eating breakfast, plan to have a snack, like a sandwich or a piece of fruit, later.

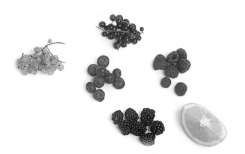

BREAKFAST SUGGESTIONS

Starting with a glass of fresh fruit juice, or a piece of fresh fruit, add any of the following:

- **Wholemeal toast** with one of the following toppings: peanut butter, a slice of lean ham, cottage cheese and reduced sugar ham, a small amount of low-fat or medium-fat cheese, or a mashed banana

Cereals with semi-skimmed milk:
- Porridge with chopped banana; 1 bowl of unsweetened muesli; 2 Shredded Wheat or Weetabix, chopped apple, raisins and walnuts; puffed rice with honey.

Cooked breakfasts:
- Wholemeal toast with grilled mushrooms and poached egg; baked beans on wholemeal toast; wholemeal toast with grilled tomatoes and lean grilled bacon; boiled egg and wholemeal toast.

Late breakfasts:
- Wholemeal and raisin muffin with a scraping of butter; low-fat yoghurt with dried apricots; wholemeal teacake with low-fat soft cheese; wholemeal scone with raisins and a little butter; sandwiches with lean ham, medium-fat cheese or a boiled egg.

LUNCH

Lunch, like breakfast, seems to be becoming less important. There is a tendency in many families, except perhaps those in which the mother or father works in the evenings or in which there are young children, to let the evening meal be the main meal of the day. Studies show that 'snack-type' lunches, such as sandwiches and fruit are just as nutritious as a cooked meal, and may even have more fibre.

What is eaten for lunch often depends on where you are. If the food that is available at school, at work, at home or in the pub is unhealthy, you may wish to bring along your own, or choose foods that have the most nutritional value, and the lowest quantities of fat and sugar.

SCHOOL OR CATERED LUNCHES

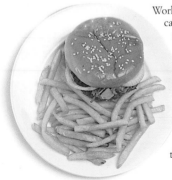

Workers who eat in a canteen, or children at school are largely at the mercy of caterers. How healthy the food will be depends on the amount and type of fat used, the amount of wholemeal products in use and the sugar added.

PACKED LUNCHES

We talk about packed lunches for children on p. 99, and many of the same principles apply for adults. Taking your own lunch to work is the most effective way of controlling what you eat at lunchtime. Besides sandwiches, try bringing a variety of salads or soups to work. If your office has a refrigerator or microwave, you can expand that list even further.

SOME LUNCH OPTIONS

Below are some examples of canteen foods that are generally healthy, as long as the cooking methods and ingredients are healthy. Try:

Fish pie
Shepherd's pie
Jacket potatoes with fillings
Cauliflower cheese
Mince and bean stew
Spaghetti
Hamburger in a wholemeal roll
Pizza
Fishfingers
Cheese salad with potato or bread
Egg salad with potato or bread
Baked beans
Vegetables
Fresh fruit
Fruit and custard
Dhal with rice

Packed lunch suggestions

Some healthy packed lunches could include:

Sandwiches
Tuna fish and salad on a wholemeal roll
A bagel with low-fat cheese and salad
Tomato and mozzarella salad with a wholemeal bap
Peanut butter on wholemeal bread
Pitta bread filled with cottage cheese and prawns
Lean roast beef or ham and salad on a wholemeal bun

Salads
Rice salad with ham, low-fat cheese, cucumber, tomato
and a light dressing
Wholemeal pasta salad, with chicken, cucumber,
sweetcorn, kidney beans and lettuce
Salad Niçoise (tuna, olives, lettuce, green beans,
tomatoes and anchovies)

THE EVENING MEAL

For many people, the evening meal is the main meal of
the day. Most effort is concentrated into preparing the
main course and vegetables may be eaten for the first
time in the day. For tips on children's meals, see pp 88-
103. Otherwise, offer them a portion of any of the
following meal suggestions.

Evening meal suggestions

- Fish pie, courgettes, carrots and green beans
- Vegetarian lasagne, cauliflower, watercress, salad,
  wholemeal rolls

- Roast chicken, rice, broad beans, leeks, carrots and cucumber salad
- Grilled fish with lemon, new potatoes, french beans and salad
- Lancashire hotpot, peas, roasted parsnips or swede
- Beef and vegetable kebab, brown rice and salad
- Grilled pork or lamb chop, fresh salad, peas, carrots and braised onions
- Chicken curry, masur dhal, cucumber raita, brown chapatti
- Any of the vegetarian meals mentioned on p. 124.

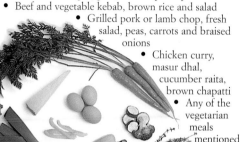

Dessert ideas
- Baked apples with raisins and yoghurt
- Fresh fruit and custard
- Frozen yoghurt with maple syrup, raisins and walnuts
- Oat-topped fruit crumbles
- Low-fat cheesecakes
- Stewed fruits
- Summer pudding
- Baked banana cooked in rum and served with yoghurt

FAST FOOD

There are a growing number of issues that relate to substances used in so-called 'fast food'.

In the UK, there have been moves to stop children eating foods rich in sugar, fat and salt, which are linked with obesity and heart disease. And there is concern that the leading burger chains are targeting children as young as two years old, making it much less likely that they will grow up eating a healthy, balanced diet.

As an odd treat, fast food should not be harmful, but used as a mainstay of any diet, it will cause health problems resulting from nutritional deficiencies. If you do give in to the odd burger or fish and chips meal, make sure you eat some fresh vegetables or salad

---

HOW HEALTHY ARE YOUR CHIPS?

If you tend to eat chips with your meal, choose thicker ones, which absorb less fat and are more nutritious. Thinner 'french fries' are more fattening. Try to avoid chips that have been fried twice. You'll need to ask about cooking methods when you order.

	Calories	Fat
1 serving (113g) fried chips	286	12.3
1 serving (113g) oven chips	212	7
Homemade chips baked with skins and a little olive oil	135	5

alongside, and cut down on your fat intake for other foods throughout the day.

When you are choosing processed foods as treats, read the labels (*see* p. 144) to ensure that the fat content isn't too high, and that the additives and preservatives are not likely to cause harm (*see* p. 142).

Nutritional content of fast food versus alternatives

• Have a quarterpounder burger and chips and you consume 791 calories with 37.1g of fat
  or
  Fill a pitta with tasty chicken morsels, tsatziki, grated carrots and chopped cucumber – 400 calories with 6g fat.

• Eat a thick-crust pepperoni pizza and you consume 940 calories with 36g fat
  or
  Make a pizza with feta cheese, half-fat mozzarella and fresh chopped vegetables, such as leeks, sweetcorn and peas – 420 calories with 9g fat.

ALTERNATIVE SNACKS

Most of us feel that a snack should require little preparation, while satisfying our desire to eat. That's one of the reasons why fast foods are so popular. All you have to do is open a packet for instant satisfaction. However, bear in mind that most commonly eaten snack foods, such as crisps, doughnuts, sausage rolls, burgers, ice cream and milkshakes, are full of fat, and usually contain little nutrition; it helps to have a supply of alternatives on hand. Keep your refrigerator and freezer full of delicious goodies that you can lay your hands on as soon as hunger strikes! Try some of the following:

- Wholegrain cereals with a low-sugar content are a good alternative to crisps.
- Pretzels are low in fat. Choose a low-salt brand.
- A bowl of fresh fruit with yoghurt, honey and some dried fruits is both satisfying and nutritious.
- Chop some fresh carrots, fresh cucumber, sugar-snap peas, mange tout and dwarf sweetcorn and dip in houmous or tsatziki.
- Make some fresh vegetable 'chips': heat a little olive oil in a baking tray. Cut sweet potato, potato, carrot, parsnip and swede into 'chip-shaped' pieces, toss in the hot oil, and roast at a high temperature until golden brown. Season with black pepper and a little sea salt and serve.
- Nuts can be fattening, but they are nutritious. Try a handful of pistachios, which take some time to

shell! Sunflower seeds are also nutritious and easy to eat.

- Offer air-popped popcorn instead of crisps and sprinkle it with a little sea salt.

- Beans on toast are always popular.

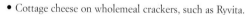

- A sandwich with lean ham or chicken and salad on a wholemeal bun.

- Any of the breakfast suggestions (*see* p. 63)!

- Low fat cheese and an apple.

- Cottage cheese on wholemeal crackers, such as Ryvita.

- A ploughman's platter, with cheese, wholemeal bread, low-sugar pickles, and raw carrots and celery.

TIPS FOR EATING OUT

Most restaurants now provide a variety of foods, and with a little careful choosing, you can eat out as healthily as you do at home. The following tips should help you to choose the healthy option, where there is a choice!

International

- Start with melon or other fruit, for a low-calorie, low-fat beginning to your meal.

- Non-creamy soups, such as carrot and fresh tomato are good options, or try a light salad with the dressing on the side.

- Choose a main course that is grilled and not served with extra fat such as a sauce.

- Avoid pastries and pies, which are bound to be high in fat.

- Try to choose foods that are high in fibre, such as a jacket potato or wholemeal bread or rice to eat with your main course.

Indian

- Indian food tends to use a lot of cream or fat in the preparation. Choose dishes that don't contain it. Tandoori cooked food, such as chicken, is a good bet.

- Rice dishes are excellent, as long as they have not been refried.

- The best breads to choose are nan and chapati. Dahl and raita are also healthy choices.

Chinese

- Chinese food can be healthy as long as it doesn't contain too much MSG (monosodium glutamate, *see* p. 142). Ask at the restaurant or takeaway which foods contain it.

- Avoid those dishes that are deep-fried, or refried.

- Try to choose a variety of dishes, including some fish, vegetables, noodles, rice and lean chicken or beef.

Italian

- Italian food can be very high in fat, but meals without heavy sauces can be nutritious. Try to stick to pasta dishes with fresh tomato or vegetable sauces.

- If you have vegetables with your meal, make sure they aren't served with butter.

- Pizza is a healthy alternative, but avoid fatty meats like pepperoni or salami, and make sure that they don't add extra cheese. A vegetarian pizza is a very nutritious meal.

Desserts

Desserts should be fruit-based, if possible, and cooked with as little sugar as possible (not always easy!)

Try fresh fruit salad, fruit marinated in liqueurs, summer pudding or baked fruits. If you plan to give in to chocolate cake at the end of the meal, make sure you balance it by eating plenty of fresh vegetables and lean meat or pasta earlier.

WHAT TO EAT, WHEN?

There are no hard and fast rules. Children, for example, may need plenty of snacks, since they may not be able to consume large quantities of food at one meal and need to boost their calorie and nutrient intake. Meals should fit your lifestyle, rather than the other way round.

- Try to avoid eating a heavy meal late at night. Not only will it make your sleep less restful, but your body will not have a chance to work it off, and much of the energy supplied will end up being laid down as fat.

- Watch out for snacking while watching television. More calories can be consumed in a single sitting than in a whole day. If you do want a snack while relaxing, put out a reasonable portion in a bowl and don't eat any more.

- Try to sit down and eat food. You'll be more aware of what you are eating. Eating on the run may be convenient, but you are less likely to manage a balanced meal, and you will probably end up feeling hungry soon after.

- Try to make at least one meal per day a 'family gathering'.

Children and eating

As any parent knows, many children are faddy eaters, others prefer to graze, and the majority would reject anything green or healthy in favour of a packet of crisps or a handful of sweets. But nutrition for children is all-important, both for their future health, their growth and development, and the choices they will make when they are old enough to plan their diets themselves.

For most people the move towards a healthy, balanced diet means eating more bread, potatoes, pasta, rice and other cereals and more fruits and vegetables, and these should form the basis of the diet of every child over five. From the ages of two to five, children need a diet that is higher in fat and lower in fibre, gradually moving towards a healthier balance.

Parents have a difficult time teaching children healthy eating habits. Advertisers bombard them with the newest junk foods and sweets and mealtimes become a battleground for many parents, as they struggle to teach the basics of healthy eating to youngsters.

CHANGING TIMES

Times have changed dramatically. Just 15 years ago, only a quarter of the processed foods now available existed. Most children were fed on a fairly balanced, if somewhat limited diet, of meat, potatoes and two vegetables, followed by a pudding, with biscuits and sweets as snacks. The vegetables may have been boiled half to death, but they still contained more nutritional value than some convenience foods.

Today, many children do not eat any fruits or vegetables (other than chips), and although they are notoriously resilient, these poor eating habits will play havoc with their growth, emotional and intellectual development, and with their later health. Heart disease is linked with a poor diet in childhood, as is osteoporosis, or brittle bone disease. If strong, healthy bone is not set down in childhood and adolescence, what hope does an elderly man or woman have?

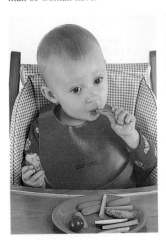

WHAT CAN WE DO?

Ensure that your children have foods from the bottom four levels of the **Food Pyramid** (*see* p. 55). If it's too much of a struggle getting them to eat Brussels sprouts and cauliflower, fruit and vegetable juices can take the place of several daily servings (*see* p. 168).

NEWBORN BABIES

Newborn babies live on milk and it is, therefore, important that your choice of milk is meeting his needs. All the studies show that it is best to breastfeed your baby, if possible. Not only does it help you to 'bond' with your newborn, but it is the most natural and nutritious food that you can offer him.

Some mothers are alarmed by the thin consistency of the milk, which looks positively anaemic next to cow's milk. Be assured, however, that it is full of the nutrients that your baby needs.

WHY BREAST MILK?

- **Nutrition:** Breast milk is designed to provide complete nourishment for a baby for several months after its birth. The mother's milk, which begins to flow a few days after childbirth as her hormones change, is a blue-white colour with a very thin consistency. If the mother is well nourished, the milk provides the baby with the proper balance of nutrition.

- **Protection from illness:** Before milk is produced the mother's breast produces **colostrum**, a deep-yellow liquid containing high levels of protein and antibodies. A newborn baby who feeds on colostrum in the first few days of life is better able to resist the bacteria and viruses that cause illness.

SOYA MILK

Soya milk is now not recommended for babies, since it contains phytooestrogens (plant oestrogen), which some experts think can damage a baby's reproductive system. Soya formula is thought to be all right.

Watch out for sugar in soya milk served to older children. Research shows that the sweeteners added to the soya to make it palatable have caused tooth decay in many children.

- **More easily digested:** The fat contained in human milk, compared with cow's milk, is more digestible for babies and allows for greater absorption of fat-soluble vitamins into the bloodstream from the baby's intestine. Calcium and other important nutrients in human milk are also better utilized by babies.

- **Less chance of allergies:** Antigens in cow's milk can cause allergic reactions in a newborn baby, whereas such reactions to human milk are rare.

- **Promotes growth:** Human milk also promotes growth, largely due to the presence of certain hormones.

- **It's free!**

BOTTLEFEEDING

Some women cannot or choose not to breastfeed. If you do feed your baby on formula, ask your midwife or doctor for advice on the best possible brand. If you have allergies in your family, you may wish to try a soya-based formula, which has no cow's milk (*see* p. 78). Alternatively, there are now pasteurized goat's milk formulas available. Read the labels carefully and compare between brands to ensure that you get a formula that offers the best nutrition.

Baby formulas

- **Advantages:** Infant formulas are very nourishing, even if they are second-best to breast milk. Someone else can feed the baby – this may be essential if you are returning to work and leaving him with a childminder.

- **Disadvantages:** Formula can prove expensive, and if you take your baby out for any length of time, you have to carry equipment and a supply of formula with you. Formula does not contain any of the protective antibodies of breast milk. Some women also find the bonding process less natural with a bottle. If you do breastfeed, give him lots of skin and eye contact, and talk to him to help intensify the feeling between you. That will also help to provide your baby with positive feelings about food and feeding.

BABIES AND TODDLERS

Your baby's main food for the first year of his life will be milk – it is easily digested and provides all the nutrition that he needs. There comes a time, however, around the four- to six-month mark (later in some cases) when he will need a little more.

WEANING

When your baby is weaned from his milk-only diet, at around four to six months, his nutritional requirements will change dramatically. First tastes will be replaced with a defined set of needs. What your toddler eats will form the backbone of his growth and development, and you will have to plan his nutritional intake carefully to ensure that he gets enough of the necessary vitamins and minerals, as well as protein, fats and carbohydrates.

BREASTFEEDING VERSUS BOTTLE FEEDING		
	Breastfeeding	**Bottle feeding**
Nutrition	Excellent	No antibodies
Expense	Free	Can be expensive
Your freedom	Have to express milk if you're going out	Anyone can feed the baby

How much does a baby need?

If your baby is happy and contented, and eating as much as he wants at each meal, then he is probably consuming the right amount of food for him. A satisfactory weight gain is also indicative of an adequate calorie intake. The approximate average daily requirements for babies aged 0 to 2 are as follows:

Age	Calories
0 to 3 months	515
3 to 6 months	695
6 to 9 months	845
9 to 12 months	945
12 to 18 months	1150
1½ to 2½ years	1350

First tastes

First foods are intended to be tastes rather than essential parts of the diet. Having said that, it is important that your baby's first foods are nutritious, and that he develops tastes for good, healthy food rather than sweets and processed foods.

> **THE BEST FIRST FOODS**
>
> • puréed apple, pear, peaches, apricots, bananas
> • puréed parsnips, swede, green beans, squash,
>   sweet potato, cauliflower, carrots, spinach, potato
>   (thinned with a little milk), peas, broccoli
> • baby rice

From about four to five months, you can begin to
introduce other cereals, such as wheat (although you
might want to wait until later, if there are any gluten
allergies in your family), oats and barley, to add some
variety.

Whichever solids you decide to offer, remember to
introduce one new food at a time, for three to four days.
It may take some time for him to become accustomed to
a new taste, and it will also give you an opportunity to
pinpoint any adverse reactions to certain foods.

Feeding your baby

Only offer a small amount to begin with – about a
teaspoonful at first, which you can increase a little each
day. When he is used to the first tastes, let him guide
you as to how much he wants to eat – within reason.
Your baby may love the taste of puréed apricots or
pears, for example, and may be happy to eat them in
large quantities.

FOODS TO AVOID:

- Egg white should be avoided until after six months old, because of the risk of allergy.

- Pork and lamb should wait until he is older, too, because they are too fatty for him to digest easily.

- Strawberries, blackcurrants and tomatoes should be avoided until after six months because they are common allergens, and they contain pips which may cause him to choke.

- Avoid food with any salt, which can put unnecessary strain on his kidneys.

- Spices can be very gradually introduced after about six or seven months.

- Sugary foods or drinks should be avoided because they can encourage a sweet tooth, and promote tooth decay.

- Cow's milk should not be offered until after at least six months. Give breast milk or formula until this time. Cow's milk is a common allergen, and the later you leave it, the more likely your baby is to take it without problems.

- Fried foods are not good for babies. Lightly steam foods when you cook them, and avoid using butter or oil.

- Nuts are also common allergens, and should not be introduced until your child is about three or four years old.

Setting up good habits

There are many things you can do during the weaning process to ensure that your baby is eating well, and that you are setting up good eating habits for later in life.

- Encourage your child to enjoy the taste of fresh fruits and vegetables. Don't be tempted to add salt, sugar or other sweeteners. Let him learn to appreciate the different tastes.

- Encourage drinking of water – plain (filtered) water should be the usual drink to quench a thirst, but diluted fruit juices can be given, too.

- Encourage chewing – most foods can be chewed by the gums to encourage strong tooth formation.

Introducing cow's milk

From about six months of age, your baby can probably drink cow's milk, but if you have allergies in your family, or he has proved to have trouble digesting it, stick to the formula you have been using throughout the first six months of his life. Your baby will need full-fat milk to provide energy as he grows bigger.

Are commercial baby foods OK?

Busy parents often rely upon commercially prepared baby foods, which can be both convenient and easy to use. There is now a wide range of organic baby foods available. Organic foods should always be chosen over cheaper, less wholesome brands if possible.

Steer clear of anything with added sugar or salt, and ensure that the ingredients are those that you would be happy to use if you were preparing the food yourself. Watch out for cheap fillers in baby food, like maltodextrin.

Introducing family foods

Try not to feed your baby on pre-prepared foods exclusively, which tend to be bland, and undoubtedly more expensive than home-prepared. Your baby needs

---

GAINING INDEPENDENCE

At some point between six and twelve months of age, your baby will want to start feeding himself, and he will attempt to explore and examine his food in much the same way as he does his toys.

Don't worry if he seems to eat odd combinations of foods, and it doesn't matter if he chooses his dessert before his main course. Let him eat what he can, and gently feed him from another bowl out of his reach, so that you are sure that something is going in!

variety, and good, wholesome food, with different tastes, textures and consistencies. If he has spent the second six months of his life eating from a jar, he may not adjust easily to family foods, when the time comes.

He needs to see that eating is a social experience, and that people sit down and eat what is put in front of them at regular times during the day. If he is fed on his own, or fed something different, on a regular basis, he is more likely to object to losing special attention when the time comes for him to join in with family meals.

If you decide to use ready-to-eat brands, don't feed him straight from the jar if you are planning to save some to use later. Store uneaten food for no more than 24 hours.

Preparing your own baby foods

If you have a liquidizer, it will be easy to prepare small quantities of whatever you are eating for your baby to try. Preparing your baby's food allows you to decide on the nutritional balance of the meal, and to choose ingredients which are fresh and healthy.

- As he grows older, you will be able to chop rather than purée his foods, and he will learn to chew.

- Don't pre-cut fruit and vegetables and leave them in water, or in air, for long periods of time, as they may lose their nutritional value.

- Don't use stock cubes or yeast extracts, which are high in salt.

- Fresh vegetables are best steamed or lightly cooked.

- To prepare for busy times, make large casseroles, or prepare large quantities of fruits and vegetables, and freeze them in small containers. You will soon build up a variety of ready-prepared meals.

- Purée baby food to a smooth consistency, adding a little milk or water if necessary.

- Remove the skin from chicken, and cut the fat off meat before cooking.

- Try to include at each meal: some brown bread, cereal or potato (carbohydrates), a little fish, chicken, milk, beans, or meat (protein) and some fresh fruits and vegetables (fibre and extra vitamins and minerals).

- Use butter and margarine sparingly.

- When reheating food, place it in a heat-resistant cup and put it in a pan of gently boiling water. If you use a microwave, take care to stir it constantly, to avoid 'hot spots'. Ensure the food has cooled sufficiently before offering it to your baby.

Meals for six- to nine-month olds

BREAKFAST

Muesli with oatmeal, ground almonds (which are hypoallergenic) and desiccated coconut

Oatmeal and apple sauce

Cheese on beans on toast

French toast

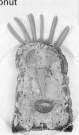

Yoghurt with bananas, fine oatmeal and dried, ready-to-eat apricots

Toast fingers with a scraping of butter or melted cheese

Diluted apple or pear juice

LUNCH

Scotch broth or vegetable broth

Lentil, creamy spinach, leek and potato, thick pea or minestrone soup

Serve with a piece of brown bread and fruit for dessert.

DINNER

Mashed beans, scrambled eggs, rice, baby-sized pasta, lean minced beef, shepherd's pie, chopped fresh vegetables and fruits, and mashed potatoes and bread.

FOODS FOR SIX-TO-NINE-MONTH OLDS

Your baby will be able to chew more, and you can now introduce food with a lumpier, or chunkier consistency. Try chopping food rather than mincing or liquidizing it, and offer small portions of your own food, if it does not contain too many seasonings.

Suitable finger foods include carrots, celery, apple (grated or in pieces), avocado, peaches, apricots, oat biscuits made without sugar or salt, cubes of cheese, and breadsticks.

FOODS FOR NINE-TO-TWELVE-MONTH-OLDS

As he nears his first birthday, your baby will be able to eat what the rest of the family is eating, but ensure that it is chopped into manageable, bite-sized pieces. You can now introduce tinned tuna, well-cooked pork, lamb with the fat cut off and drained, and some fruits such as oranges and raspberries, which were not appropriate in early babyhood.

He will be able to pick up a broccoli 'tree' and try to eat it himself, or gnaw at a Brussels sprout. Try to include some foods that require feeding (which he will be learning to do himself) and others that he will be able to pick up and eat himself.

All foods should be minced until your child is happy with lumps and then the pieces can gradually be cut larger when he is able to chew properly.

Meals for nine- to twelve-month-olds

Scrambled eggs with cheese and spinach

Wholemeal bread with beans and sliced boiled egg

Pressure-cooked cheesy vegetables

Cheese and tomato pizza with sweetcorn, peas and pineapple on top

Simple salmon salad: cucumber, tinned salmon, mashed into natural unsweetened yoghurt

Tuna pasta: baby pasta with a light white sauce, peas, carrot, spinach and grated cheese on top

Lamb's liver and vegetable casserole (use marmite in boiling water to make the stock)

Chicken casserole (tomato juice for stock); add mixed herbs and vegetables and serve with rice

Mince and parsnip bake, with finely chopped peas, carrots and celery in a tomato juice broth

Macaroni cheese with spinach

Spaghetti bolognaise

DESSERTS

Puréed pear mixed with natural yoghurt

Apple fool: fromage frais mixed with puréed apple

Rice pudding with sultanas (use pasteurized honey instead of sugar in the mix)

Baked peach custard

FOODS FOR TODDLERS

From the age of around two, your child should be eating a family meal and the rules for adults apply, although portion sizes wil be smaller (see below). The four main groups of food, which form the basis of the **Food Pyramid** (see p. 55) will provide almost all the nutrients he or she needs.

- Try not to offer more than one serving per day of biscuits, cakes, puddings, sweets or icecream.

- Offer your child lots of fresh water to drink between meals to help the body work more efficiently. Avoid sweet drinks and only offer fruit juices with meals.

- Try to ensure that your child eats at least two hot, nutritious meals a day. If your child will eat cold

---

FAMILY PORTIONS

In a family of two adults and three children aged 12 months, 9 years and 12 years, the baby will eat half as much food as his father or mother, and the two older children will probably be eating as much as, or more than, their parents.

Huge appetites at a young age are common but can sometimes catch parents unawares! Serving a larger portion of food to Dad than to the 12-year-old may help explain obesity in adults, and the seemingly bottomless appetites of children, particularly when they reach puberty.

vegetables, such as salads, cold sweetcorn, cucumber, etc., you can provide nutritious meals that are cold.

- Stick to the healthy eating guidelines, ensuring that your child is getting enough servings of all the important nutrients.

FUSSY EATERS

You may be very worried if your child refuses to eat or is a 'faddy' or 'picky' eater. Try to remember that it is extremely rare for a child to actually starve himself. Children will eat enough to keep going. Try not to worry unless your child is clearly not gaining weight, or is obviously unwell.

It may be that your child is picking up your own feelings about food. Perhaps you're a dieter or have a weight problem, or maybe you just see healthy eating as a very important goal. If your child is sensing your anxiety it may be that mealtimes have become an ideal time to get attention. Try to take a step back and consider whether your child's eating habits really are a problem.

PRACTICAL ADVICE FOR PARENTS OF FUSSY EATERS

- Ask another adult, whom your child likes, to eat with you. Sometimes a child will eat for, say, a grandparent without any fuss. It may be only one meal out of many, but it could break a habit.

- Children often prefer to eat when you eat – especially when they are toddlers.

- One day your child will hate something and a month later they'll love it – bear with them.

- Don't force your child to eat or to finish everything on their plate 'to please Mummy'. This can make children feel insecure.

- Don't get trapped into giving your child a sweet treat after an uneaten meal.

- Don't leave meals until your child is overtired or too hungry.

- For very fussy eaters, nutritious snacks between meals can help to make sure they meet their needs (*see* **Healthy snacks** p. 95).

- If you know other children of the same age who are good eaters, ask them to tea. A good example sometimes works, as long as you don't go on about how good the other children are.

- If your child refuses food or just picks at his food for a long time, call an end to the meal. Do it calmly and not in anger, no matter what time and effort you've put into the cooking.

- Put less food on your child's plate and praise your child for eating even a little.

- Try to make meals enjoyable and not just about eating.

- Your child may just be a naturally slow eater, and so be patient.

TEACHING HEALTHY EATING HABITS

- Keep healthy snacks in the refrigerator, and encourage children to help themselves to fruit between meals.

- Practise what you preach: if you constantly reach for a bag of crisps, your children will too.

- Only purchase foods that you want your children to eat. There is no point in keeping supplies of junk food to save for special treats. The temptation may be too tantalizing, and there will be an unnatural association between goodies and normal eating habits.

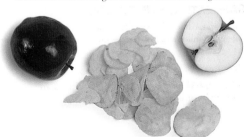

HEALTHY SNACKS FOR CHILDREN

- fresh and dried fruit
- raw vegetables like carrots, courgettes,
    sweet peppers
- natural yoghurt with fresh fruit
- chunks of cheese
- unsweetened breakfast cereals (dry or with milk)
- bread
- popcorn
- bread sticks

- Don't use junk foods or chocolates as a bribe to encourage your children to finish their meal.

- Encourage your children to help you with the cooking. Vary meals and make an effort to present them in an attractive style.

SAFE EATING FOR CHILDREN

Even the most wholesome food may not be suitable for a baby or child, and it is important to learn what foods are and are not safe.

Here are some of the main issues:

- Fatty meats like pork or fattier cuts of beef are difficult for children to digest.

- Cured meat like bacon, ham and salami may be fatty, and both these and smoked fish contain preservatives called nitrates which have been banned from baby and toddler foods.

- Fish is a great food for children, but you must watch out for small bones which can become lodged in their throats.

- Watch the salt content – salt places an enormous strain on children's kidneys, which have not developed enough to cope. Avoid mineral water for under-5s, as it may have a high salt content.

HEALTHY FAST FOOD

- fruit and vegetables
- wholemeal bread or toast
- baked beans
- baked potatoes with tuna, baked beans, cheese, roasted vegetables, or tinned sweetcorn
- fish fingers and frozen fish generally – but grilled or baked rather than fried.
- tinned fish
- tinned tomatoes
- natural yoghurt with honey and fruit
- boiled eggs
- pasta with tomato sauce
- vegetable 'chips' (see p. 70)

FOOD HYGIENE

- Encourage your children to wash their hands before they eat anything. Good habits are established early. Children are in contact with a wide range of bacteria and viruses, both through play outside, with animals and with other children. It's important that these are not ingested through contact with food.

- If children are outside and eating with their hands, teach them to hold the food with a paper napkin to avoid the spread of germs.

- Avoid unpasteurized dairy products, soft cheeses, cook-chilled convenience foods and soft eggs. Goat's and ewe's milk are generally unpasteurized.

- Cut down on brightly coloured or highly sweetened foods and snacks, especially sweets and soft drinks,

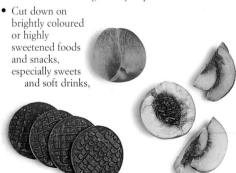

which contain colourings, flavourings and
preservatives that can cause health problems in
children.

- E numbers to avoid include: E102, E104, E107,
E110, E120, E122, E123, E124, E127, E128, E131,
E132, E133, E150, E151, E154, E155, E160B, E210,
E211, E220, E250, E251, E320 and E321. These
additives have been linked with behavioural problems
in children (*see* p. 105).

BREAKFAST

With children taking packed lunches, or eating school
dinners, you may have little control over what they eat
in the daytime, and they may feel too tired, after an
active day, to eat a proper meal after school. You do
have some control over breakfast, and it is worth
waking up early to ensure that they get a good,
nutritious meal. Studies show that children who have a
balanced, healthy breakfast, which includes some
protein, can perform better at school, and have greater
concentration skills.

Try:

- fresh fruit with a
dollop of yoghurt,
fresh honey and
muesli
- a hard-boiled egg
with toast and a glass
of fresh orange juice.

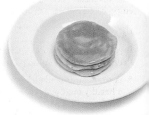

- American-style pancakes with fresh maple syrup (pancakes contain flour, eggs and milk, all of which are healthy options) and a glass of juice.

- a healthy cereal, with no added sugar, such as cornflakes, Weetabix or porridge

- wholemeal toast with yeast extract, melted cheese or peanut butter (over the age of three or four), and a glass of fresh juice

- French toast, using wholemeal bread, and a glass of fresh juice

- Welsh rarebit, with a thin layer of tomatoes under the cheese

LUNCHBOXES

You can also help your child by ensuring he eats a healthy, balanced meal at lunchtime. If a hot meal is served at school, encourage him to eat 'a green and a red or orange vegetable' with every meal, and to choose fruit at least three times a week. Some families set a 'chips once a week' rule, where the child can have chips with his meal. Let him choose the day, and he'll feel empowered rather than ruled.

PACKED LUNCHES

If you make a lunchbox for your child, choose foods that are easy to eat and look tempting.

- A wholemeal sandwich with cheese and cucumber is a healthy option, or try tuna and sweetcorn in a wholemeal pitta.

- If your child is a grazer, chop up pieces of fruits and vegetables, and give him a dip in a small plastic container.
- String pieces of fresh fruit on a kebab stick and provide a tub of yoghurt for dipping.

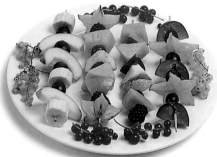

- Most supermarkets sell small apples, pears and bananas that are the perfect size for a lunchbox, and a handful of grapes, a low-sugar muesli bar and a yoghurt make the meal complete.
- The odd small chocolate biscuit or bag of crisps won't matter, as long as your children eat plenty of fresh vegetables, whole grains, fruit and dairy produce, with some meat or other protein foods.
- Try a hard-boiled egg, some rice crackers spread with yeast extract or cheese, and a selection of fruits such

as plums, nectarines, strawberries, or anything else in season.

- A chunk of wholemeal bread, with the makings of a sandwich – lean ham, salad, cheese, chicken or fish – may be more tempting than a soggy sandwich. Let him make his own at school, or eat the bits separately. Whatever way he does it, you'll know that he's had a balanced meal.

- Cold pizza or a cold chicken leg are healthy options for lunchtimes.

- Send fresh diluted fruit juices in a thermos, or one of the pure fruit juice boxes if the price isn't too prohibitive. Hot food can also be sent in a thermos.

- Talk to your child's school about the way they eat lunch. Ensure that they are encouraged to eat the healthy bits of the lunch before the crisps or 'treat'. Ask them to send the lunchbox home unemptied, so you get an idea of what has or hasn't been eaten.

- Ensure the school allows time for the children to wash their hands before lunch.

- Make sure you keep the lunchboxes clean and dry between use. If you make your lunches in advance, keep the lunchbox in the refrigerator until your child sets off for school.

- Invest in an insulated lunchbox, with cooling blocks to keep food fresh.

ADOLESCENTS

Adolescence is a time of great physical and emotional change, and it is also a period in which your control over your child's diet may be severely tested. A wholesome, healthy diet is crucial to both the physical and intellectual development of an adolescent, and yet peer pressure may make this difficult.

The 'growth spurt' occurs at different ages. For boys it is between 12 and 19; for girls it is between 10 and 15. During this growth spurt the body needs more calories than at any other period, except infancy.

The main recommendations for adolescents are:

- eat a healthy, varied diet
- cut down on fat, sugar and salt
- increase the intake of fibre.

FAST FOOD

Diets that include a large proportion of fast foods (*see* p. 68) can be deficient in some nutrients, particularly vitamin C, iron, folic acid and riboflavin. Fast foods also tend to be high in calories, fat (particularly saturated fat), salt and sugar, and low in fibre.

WHAT DO ADOLESCENTS NEED?

The adolescent diet should mirror the diet of his parents, with special attention paid to fibre, iron and protein.

- **Protein** is needed for growth during this important time, so if your child follows the burgeoning trend towards vegetarianism, make sure that he is getting enough vegetable proteins (*see* p. 39).

- Teenagers should try to increase the amount of **fibre** in their diet by eating wholemeal and high-fibre foods. Sandwiches on wholemeal bread are nutritious, as are baked beans, nuts, dried fruits and wholemeal breakfast cereals. As many wholemeal products are also higher in iron than refined varieties, increasing fibre intake also ensures that iron intake is increased.

- **Iron** is needed both for the development of new muscle tissue and to cope with increased haemoglobin demands. Iron is particularly important during menstruation so girls who are still growing when their periods start need to have plentiful supplies. Iron-rich foods include meats, leafy green vegetables and dried fruits.

Calories

Calorie needs will be completely dependent upon your child's size, the rate at which he is growing, and how active he is. You can expect most adolescents to eat between 2000 and 3000 calories each day. The same principle applies as for younger children's eating habits: as long as your child is growing well, and not having any developmental problems, the amount of food consumed can be dictated by how hungry he is!

WHEN FOOD BECOMES A PROBLEM

When your child's behaviour or health suffers, you may be right to question his diet. Some illnesses may be caused by food allergies or intolerances. The focus on food, diet and being slim and healthy has also put youngsters, particularly adolescent girls, under enormous pressure to be thinner than they should be.

FOOD ALLERGIES

More is now known about allergies in small children and they appear to run in families. Here are the facts:

- Some of the most common food allergens include cow's milk, chocolate, citrus fruit, grapes, wheat, oranges, cheese, eggs, peanuts and maize. Symptoms of a food allergy can include rashes, stomach aches, headaches and hyperactivity.

- Common allergens should be introduced one at a time in childhood, and only after your child has reached his first birthday (avoid some of the worst offenders, such as peanuts, until they are three or four). If symptoms appear, such as lethargy, unexplained tummy ache, rashes or just general malaise, cut out the food in question and wait a few months before trying it again.

OBESITY

If your child is fat, it is important to realize that they need to be highly motivated in order to lose weight. Nagging will not make things any better, nor will making jokes about their size. If food has become something other than a source of energy or pleasure, you might need to talk things over with your doctor.

People who have been fat as children are more likely to run a risk of developing the early stages of heart disease, and their ability to control blood sugar can be damaged.

HYPERACTIVITY

Some experts believe that there is a link between hyperactivity and diet. Causes could include food allergy or intolerance, heavy metal toxicity, sugar sensitivity, candida, food additive sensitivity and deficiencies of Zinc, B vitamins, Magnesium, Chromium and essential fatty acids. Consult your doctor if you are worried about your child's behaviour.

What can you do?

- Try to avoid dieting, which can make food into an issue, and make him long for the foods that everyone else is eating. Change your family diet to one that is healthier overall, with fewer fats, and more complex carbohydrates, and the excess weight should decline gradually.

- If you have an adolescent who is overweight, you can talk about their feelings if the right opportunity arises. Do what you can to encourage them and strengthen their motivation.

- On a practical level, you will need to make changes in their eating habits at home, cutting out snacks that are high in fat and sugar and, therefore, calories.

- Crash dieting is not advisable. It is easy to regain lost weight once the diet is over, and to fall into a pattern of dieting, followed by weight gain, followed by further dieting.

- The aim should be to establish a way of eating that is nutritious and satisfying and can become a lifelong habit. Together with extra exercise, this should be enough to get down to a healthy weight. Above all, the overweight adolescent who is trying to eat sensibly needs all the support that the family can offer.

EATING DISORDERS

There are many theories about what causes anorexia and bulimia, and certainly the sufferers are mostly, but not always, adolescent girls. If a young person behaves in a way that suggests they are anorexic or bulimic (*see* below) tell them about your concern, and seek help as soon as possible.

Getting help

The family doctor can recommend associations that can offer help and information (*see also* p. 192). Changing eating habits can be a lengthy process and can involve the whole family. Parents feel bewildered and guilty, but it is very important to realize that the condition is not their fault. Living with an anorexic or bulimic calls for love and patience and family members need to share their feelings and to listen to one another.

SOME COMMON SIGNS OF AN EATING DISORDER INCLUDE:

- never being content with their weight loss
- setting lower and lower weight targets
- suffering from a totally unrealistic body image
- obsession with perfection
- denial that there is a problem
- secretive behaviour and excuse-making
- ritualistic eating
- signs of purging, including laxatives and vomiting
- unusual eating habits which include regular binges that are not reflected by any weight gain

---

Special needs

One criticism of doctors is that they treat all of us alike, prescribing the same dietary rules for all. It is clear that we all need food to survive, and that regular, healthy eating will promote good health, but we are all different, and what is a good way of eating for one person may not be for another. There are, however, very general 'rules' that may be applied to specific age groups, for example, or to different sexes.

Our needs change at different stages of our lives, and according to our lifestyles. Women, for example, tend to need more iron while they are in their fertile years, and calcium is important to prevent osteoporosis in older people and to help form strong bones and teeth in children. Smokers need to get more vitamin C, and anyone who drinks alcohol on a regular basis should make sure that the B vitamins are adequately represented in their diets.

A good healthy diet, following the **Food Pyramid** (*see* p. 55), should ensure that you get enough of the nutrients you need for good health. But in cases of ill health, and at certain times of life, you may need more of some nutrients, especially vitamins and minerals.

Certain groups of the population are particularly vulnerable to nutritional deficiencies, including pregnant or breastfeeding women, those on weight-loss diets, children, adolescents and the elderly.

YOUR BODY WILL MAKE CLEAR WHEN EVEN SMALL NUTRITIONAL DEFICIENCIES ARE PRESENT	
SYMPTOM	POSSIBLE DEFICIENCY
Constipation	B-complex
Diarrhoea	Niacin (B3) and vitamin K
Eye problems	Vitamin A
Fatigue	Zinc, Iron, vitamins A, B, C, D
Hair problems	Vitamin B12, B6 and Selenium
Infections	Vitamin A, B-complex, Biotin, Calcium, Potassium
Muscle cramps	Vitamin B1, Biotin, Sodium, vitamin D
Nervousness	B6, B12, B3, Magnesium, vitamin C
Skin problems	Vitamin A, B-complex, Biotin, Copper

WOMEN

Women have clearly defined nutritional needs that change as they age and throughout their various cycles. Many women can be deficient in the basic vitamins and minerals, partly because their needs have not been met with decent food and balanced meals, partly because of eating low-calorie diets in a slimming programme, and partly because of the increased stress placed on women who try to juggle a family, a home and often a career, without increasing their nutritional resources.

Women who take the Pill will require different supplements from women who are experiencing the menopause. Breastfeeding and pregnant women have massive nutritional requirements (*see* pp 111-15), and menstruating women are different again.

CALORIE NEEDS

On average, women will need the following number of calories at different stages of their lives:

Young adults	2150
Pregnant	2400
Breastfeeding	2700
Middle-aged	1900 (2500 if very active)
Over 75	1680

WHAT WOMEN NEED

- Women with PMS should increase their intake of vitamin B6 (found in avocados, bananas, fish and eggs). If a supplement is necessary, you'll need about 25mg per day. Take an evening primrose capsule. Take chromium at 200mcg daily, and add fish oils, at 2,000–3,000mg per day.

- Post-menopausal women will need extra antioxidants (found in bright-coloured fruits and vegetables), as well as increased calcium (600–1,200mg per day). Calcium-rich foods include dairy products and leafy green vegetables. Boron can help to protect against osteoporosis.

- Women with a heavy monthly blood loss may need an iron supplement, particularly if they are fitted with an IUD. Eat plenty of iron-rich foods (see p. 51), including meats and leafy green vegetables. If you do need to take a supplement, take 10 to 15mg daily, either by itself or with vitamin C for maximum absorption.

- Women suffering from stress should take ginseng to help increase energy levels. Make sure you get lots of B vitamins (found in whole grains, among other things), to keep your nerves healthy!

PREGNANCY AND PRECONCEPTION

During the preconceptual period and pregnancy there is an enormous responsibility to eat well, to ensure the health and safety of the unborn baby. It is important to ensure that you eat foods from all the main levels of the **Food Pyramid** (see p. 55), and cut out anything that may have a detrimental effect on your baby, such as foods containing additives, or foods that may pose a health risk, such as uncooked eggs.

Experts recommend that a good multi-vitamin and mineral tablet should be taken alongside a healthy diet. Folic acid is particularly important (see p. 112). Don't overuse supplements in pregnancy; taking too much of any vitamin or mineral can upset the balance, and some vitamins and minerals are toxic in large doses.

WHAT YOU NEED

- Three to six months before you intend to conceive, you should start taking at least 400 mcg of folic acid daily to help prevent birth defects, such as spina bifida. Folic acid forms an important part of preconceptual care. Continue to take a folic acid supplement throughout pregnancy, and eat foods that are rich in this important vitamin, such as leafy green vegetables and wholegrains.

- Make sure that you do not get more than 10,000 iu of vitamin A each day, which could cause birth defects in your unborn baby. Take vitamin A as betacarotene, which is safer. Better still, ensure that you get all the vitamin A you need from your diet. Good sources include bright-coloured fruits and vegetables. Avoid liver.

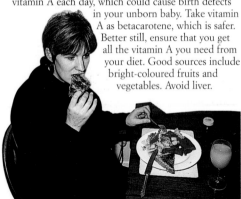

- Get plenty of Zinc. Good sources include seeds, nuts and wholegrains.

- Eat 6 to 9 portions of fresh fruits and vegetables a day – organic if you can get them, because organic produce can have up to 100 percent more nutritional value than commercially grown varieties.

WHAT TO AVOID

- Try not to binge too much on a single food. Children can be born allergic to substances their mothers ate frequently during pregnancy, and peanuts appear to be a common culprit.

TIPS FOR A HEALTHY PREGNANCY

Avoid	Add
Soft cheeses	Folic acid
Cook-chilled meals	Fresh fruit
Raw eggs	Fresh vegetables
Soft-boiled eggs	Wholemeal breads
Peanuts	Seeds, nuts (not peanuts)
Liver	Brown rice
Unwashed fruits and vegetables	Whole grains
Coffee and caffeine-containing drinks.	
Alcohol	
Overheated cooking oil	
Charred or barbecued foods	

- Cook-chilled meals and ready-cooked chicken should be safe if they are heated until they are piping hot but you may want to avoid them until after your baby is born.

- Toxoplasmosis can be carried on unwashed fruits and vegetables or undercooked meat, so make sure the produce is washed and the meat well done.

- Alcohol is best avoided during the first five to six months of pregnancy, although some experts believe that a drink in late pregnancy will help to relax you and will do no harm to your growing baby.

- Overheated cooking oil and charred, barbecued foods can interfere with healthy conception and birth.

BREASTFEEDING MOTHERS

Breastfeeding women must continue the good eating habits of pregnancy. You are likely to feel hungrier and will need to eat more to ensure that you are receiving adequate calories and nutrition to feed a baby and remain in good health.

Use the **Food Pyramid** (*see* p. 55) as your guide, and make sure you are getting all the required elements. If you are hungry, listen to your body and eat! You'll need about 600 more calories per day than you did before you were pregnant.

For 600 calories, you could have a variety of nutritious snacks, including two toasted bagels with low-fat cream cheese and an apple; four pieces of toast lightly spread

---

TIPS FOR HEALTHY EATING WHILE BREASTFEEDING

- Try to eat three good meals, as well as snacks in between, to keep your blood sugar levels steady.

- Avoid dieting while breastfeeding. Your energy levels will flag and you will find it difficult to supply your baby with enough milk. Also, your nutritional needs and those of your baby could be compromised.

- Focus on good eating habits while feeding your baby, and take some gentle exercise; you are more likely to lose the weight safely.

- Ensure that you take a good vitamin and mineral supplement, with iron and Zinc, to prevent possible deficiencies.

---

with yeast extract; several pieces of fruit and three pots of yoghurt; or two tuna sandwiches with salad on wholemeal bread, and low-fat mayonnaise.

MEN

Studies show that men are much less interested in their nutritional status than women, and are far less likely to supplement in order to meet their nutritional needs. Increased stress levels and the effects of pollution in our modern society have, however, caused some nutritional deficiencies which may need to be met with supplements and/or an improved diet.

What You Need

The daily needs of men should be adequately met by following the **Food Pyramid** (*see* p. 55). Men still drink more alcohol and smoke more than women, and will need to take extra vitamins and minerals to help prevent long-term damage to their bodies.

- Men who are athletic will need extra magnesium, at 200 mg per day, and a good antioxidant preparation.

- Men who have been diagnosed as suffering from prostate enlargement should take extra Vitamin B-complex, up to 50 mg

CALORIE NEEDS

On average, men will need the following number of calories at different stages of their lives:

Young adults	2510 (3350 if very active)
Middle-aged	2400 (3350 if very active)
Over 75	2150

daily, with 15 to 20mg of zinc.

- Men with a reduced sperm count will benefit from extra vitamin C (1000 mg spread over three doses on a daily basis), and extra zinc (15–20 mg daily).

- Because heart disease is still more common in men, supplements to ensure a healthy heart will be useful. It is recommended that all men take a garlic supplement daily, and get plenty of antioxidants (found in bright-coloured fruits and vegetables) to help prevent oxidative damage to the heart.

THE ELDERLY

The degenerative effects of ageing often take their toll, with a host of chronic and acute health conditions becoming part of daily life. However, by using supplements and the tools of nutrition to best effect, our later years can be more fruitful and healthy.

Diet is important at any age, and it is vital that we do not lose interest in the food we eat, and its role in our body as we age. If the amount eaten declines substantially, health may be affected. A decline in food intake can be associated with a number of factors, such as poor health, a recent bereavement resulting in living alone, and having to cook for one.

Elderly people who are chronically ill are most likely to be at risk of nutritional deficiency. Pain, handicap, drug use and badly fitting dentures can make getting and eating an adequate diet very difficult.

HEALTHY EATING TIPS FOR THE ELDERLY

- Cut down on fats, and use olive oil, which is the healthiest oil, and is associated with longevity and reduced cholesterol and heart disease.

- Ensure that your teeth are cared for, and that if you have dentures they are well-fitting. Studies show that poor chewing is a cause of malnutrition in some elderly people. Chewing food produces saliva, which helps to keep your mouth healthy, and stimulates the taste buds. If you can't taste your food, you are much less likely to find it interesting.

- Try to find time to eat with a friend, or take a sandwich to the local park. Loneliness and depression in old age can lead to self-neglect.

- Although the protein requirements diminish with age, as lean muscle tissue is reduced, so does the ability to digest and absorb food. Protein intake therefore needs to be adequate.

- Fibre is increasingly important as we age. Constipation can be a problem as the digestive system becomes less efficient in older people, particularly if there is inadequate exercise. Rather than using bran or laxatives, it is best to consume a diet that is high in fibre (*see* p. 34). If bran or wholemeal cereal is not enough, try plenty of fresh fruit juices and increase your intake of water.

- Fresh fruits and vegetables are an important source of antioxidants, and more than ever it is important to include these in your daily diet. If it is impossible to eat foods raw, then lightly steam or stew them and mix them with something soft like couscous (for vegetables) or oatmeal (for fruit).

- Vitamin C is required more and more as we age and our immune system becomes more vulnerable to infection. If it is difficult to chew fresh foods, several glasses of fruit or vegetable juices will help to keep levels up. Kiwi fruits, which are easy to eat and fairly soft, are very high in vitamin C, and certainly as affordable as oranges. Other good sources of vitamin C include strawberries, broccoli, cauliflower, raspberries and blackberries.

- Vitamin D is needed to transport calcium from the blood to the bones and back again. As the majority of our vitamin D comes from sunlight, try to sit in the summer sun whenever possible (with a suitable sunscreen). Alternatively, you may wish to consider a vitamin D supplement.

Vegetarians

The number of vegetarians in the Western world is rising all the time, and recent estimates indicate that at least 10 percent of the population embrace some form of vegetarianism, even if it is part time. Ethical and religious considerations have traditionally led people to choose a vegetarian diet, but in recent years, health and ecological issues have become important.

TYPES OF VEGETARIAN

The term vegetarianism is often used quite loosely, and some people call themselves vegetarian yet still eat white meats, such as fish, shellfish and chicken. Vegans eat a range of plant foods, but no products of animal origin. Lactovegetarians eat dairy food such as cheese and yoghurt, and drink milk. This diet, with the addition of eggs, is also eaten by ovo-lactovegetarians.

IS A VEGETARIAN DIET HEALTHIER?

If saturated fats, such as cheese and full-fat milk, are kept to a minimum, most vegetarians do have a lower blood cholesterol level (see pp 27-8), and a higher intake of fibre (nearly 30–50 percent higher than the average meat-eater). This reduces the risk of cardiovascular and digestive disease, among other things. Vegetarians are also generally less obese than meat-eaters, and suffer from fewer vitamin and mineral deficiencies, provided they eat a varied diet.

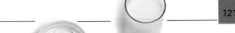

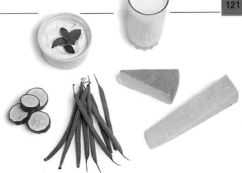

PROTEIN

The stumbling block for many vegetarians, however, is protein intake. A vegetarian diet should contain a variety of foods, such as cereals, beans, nuts, pulses and vegetables, which ensures a good balance of proteins and other nutrients. These foods should predominate in the diet (particularly if fewer dairy products are consumed) to ensure that adequate quantities of protein are available for the processes of the body, including the rebuilding of the body's tissues.

IRON

Lack of iron can also be a problem for vegetarians, particularly for teenagers. Increased amounts of beans, pulses, nuts, dried fruit or wholegrain cereals should help to overcome this problem, and fresh fruit and vegetables will provide the vitamin C necessary for the iron to be absorbed.

VEGETARIAN CHILDREN

Children can thrive on a properly balanced vegetarian diet, but it is important that they get a higher percentage of protein and calories relative to their body weight. A diet that includes pulses at least once a day, wholemeal bread or cereals two or three times a day and a pint of milk or its equivalent in dairy foods such as cheese, yoghurt or soya milk, plus the necessary fruits and vegetables (5–7 servings a day is recommended for children), will contain more than enough protein and vitamins and minerals.

Calories

It is also important to ensure that they get enough calories, since vegetarian foods tend to be bulkier and to satisfy the appetite more readily. If your child eats lots of pasta, for instance, ensure that he gets plenty of a nutritious sauce alongside, both to bump up the calorie and nutrition intake, and to ensure that he isn't filling up on one type of food only. If your child continues to gain weight and grow normally, you can be assured that his diet is satisfactory.

CHANGING TO A VEGETARIAN DIET

If you are thinking of changing to a vegetarian diet, you'll need to ensure that you get enough of each of the important food groups. There are many vegetarian products now available in supermarkets, but the same caution must be exercised as with any convenience foods. Read the label for fat content and E-numbers (*see* p. 144).

Here are some guidelines for adopting a vegetarian diet:

- Use beans and pulses to replace meat and meat products
- Eat plenty of high-fibre foods, such as brown rice, wholemeal bread, wholemeal pasta and wholemeal breakfast cereals.
- Remember to include some salads in your diet.
- Vegetables that are cooked for a long time lose most of their folic acid.
- Use only the minimum of oil or other fats when frying.
- Try to avoid high-fat foods, such as hard cheese and full-fat milk.
- Try not to rely entirely on convenience foods. Fresh foods are more likely to provide you with the extra vitamins, minerals and other elements of nutrition that you need.

SUGGESTIONS FOR VEGETARIAN MEALS

Most vegetarian meals can be frozen, so it is a good idea to double or even triple the quantities and keep some meals in the freezer as standbys. The following meals are both healthy and, with a green salad, a wholegrain roll and a piece of fruit (dried or fresh) for dessert, balanced.

Try:

Wholemeal pancakes stuffed with stir-fried vegetables, vegetables in a low-fat cheese sauce, or ratatouille

Homemade vegetable soups, such as carrot and coriander, potato and leek, spinach, tomato and basil or a hearty vegetable soup with pulses and dried vegetables

Vegetable lasagne

Wholemeal quiche

Stuffed vegetables

Risotto with fresh sautéed vegetables

Marinated tofu, with stir-fried vegetables and rice

Vegetarian stew, moussaka, goulash or curry

Mushroom burgers, or other substitutes, on a wholemeal bun

Nut roasts, or nut or bean rissoles

Baked beans on toast

VEGANS

A vegan diet contains even more bulk than a vegetarian one, and it is therefore more difficult to ensure that you get the required nutritional elements, and calories. The most common nutrients lacking in a vegan diet are calcium, Vitamin D and Vitamin B12.

Vitamin B12 is found mainly in animal products, and also in miso, tempeh, brewer's yeast and soya milks that have been fortified. The latter foods cannot be eaten in large enough quantities to provide the required daily intake, so it is recommended that all vegans take a vitamin B12 supplement. Children should be given fortified soya milk regularly (*see* p. 78) as well as a supplement.

Calcium is found in a variety of non-dairy foods, but it is important to ensure that these foods are eaten regularly. High-calcium foods include broccoli, soya beans, almonds, tofu, soya milk (or soya yoghurt and cheese), dried fruits and dark green vegetables.

Vitamin D can be synthesized by the body when it receives adequate sunlight, and sunscreens do not hamper this action.

SPECIAL NEEDS

Our nutritional needs also change according to our level of health, and our lifestyles. The following chart will help you see what nutrients may be inadequately supplied in your diet.

If you	Make sure you get enough
Smoke	**Vitamin C**. Smoking strips the body of vitamin C, among other things. In fact, studies show that each cigarette increases your vitamin C requirements by 25mg! That's half an orange's worth of vitamin C. You'll also need to eat plenty of foods that are high in antioxidants (*see* p. 49), which can help to protect against some of the negative effects of smoking on the body.
Drink alcohol	**B vitamins**. B vitamins are stripped from the body when we drink too much, or too regularly. Ensure that you eat plenty of foods rich in these vitamins.
Have a cold or flu	**Vitamin C** and **zinc**. Studies show that vitamin C, at one to two grams daily during the course of a cold can reduce the number of days a cold lasts. Zinc should be taken alongside, and at the first hint of a cold.

If you	Make sure you get enough
Are an athlete	**Vitamin E**. Vitamin E is recommended for all endurance athletes and anyone performing strenuous activity for long periods of time. You'll also need to ensure that you get plenty of iron.
Are overweight	**Chromium** and **fibre**. Chromium helps to balance blood sugar, and if you find that you have cravings for food between meals, and feel faint, you may need to eat more Chromium-rich foods (*see* p. 51). Fibre encourages proper digestion and helps you to feel fuller.
Are tired all the time	**B vitamins**, **iron** and **vitamin C**. The B-complex vitamins help the body to metabolize energy. If you are tired all the time, you may not be getting enough. Too little iron in the diet can cause anaemia. Be sure to eat plenty of iron-rich foods. Vitamin C helps to keep the immune system functioning. If you are tired for no apparent reason, you may be fighting a low-grade virus. Eat plenty of foods rich in vitamin C to help fight it off.

Choosing and preparing foods

Choosing the right foods is the first step towards a healthy diet. The next step is learning the best ways to store, prepare and cook your healthy foods.

FRESH IS BEST

Fresh foods are always the best first option. It is important to ensure that the food you are buying is fresh at the point of sale, and that you eat it while it is still fresh.

Foods that have sat for any length of time on a supermarket shelf, or in transit on the way to the supermarket, are likely to have lost some of their nutritional value. If you are concerned, you should ask how fresh food is and where it has come from.

INTERNATIONAL FOOD

These days there is often little difference in what is available on the supermarket shelves, whether it's summer, autumn, winter or spring. Apples may not be ripe locally – so we simply fly them in from New Zealand, Chile or South Africa. Avocados may not grow in this country, but we can ship them halfway around the world. Similarly, we are offered mangoes from India, mangetout peas from Kenya and new potatoes from Cyprus.

Increasingly, varieties of fruits and vegetables are picked
for their size, ability to travel long distances and for
their shelf-life, rather than for their taste.

Is it a good thing?

Quite apart from the fact that a great deal of fuel is
required to fly these foods around the world, and that
our local varieties are diminishing, food travelling long
distances simply cannot be as healthy as food picked
around the corner, at the correct stage of ripeness, and
purchased by the consumer on the same day or shortly
after. With every day that passes after picking, fresh
fruits and vegetables are reduced in nutritional value.

WHY EAT LOCAL, IN-SEASON PRODUCE?

- Local produce is more likely to have been harvested
  recently.
- Local produce will not
  be contaminated
  with chemicals
  that have been
  banned over
  here.
- Local
  produce
  will not
  introduce
  new bacteria,
  viruses and other
  'bugs'.

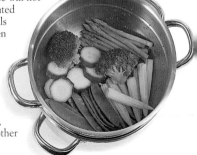

CHOOSING FOOD

FRESH FOODS

- Wherever they come from, fruits and vegetables should look fresh and undamaged.

- Leaves should be crisp, root vegetables firm, with the skin unbroken.

- Fruits like melons should smell ripe but not too sweet, and should be firm to the touch.

- Food doesn't have to be uniformly sized to be healthy; organic food comes in all different shapes, shades and sizes, which is the way that fresh vegetables grow naturally (*see* pp 158-9).

- Ready-prepared salads and chopped vegetables are inferior to their fresh, uncut counterparts, but if you don't have time for much food preparation, and are unlikely to eat anything fresh unless it is prepared for you, then these are a good buy. Watch out, however, for any signs of age, such as browning edges on lettuce, dried-out vegetables, and excess moisture in the package.

TINNED FOODS

Tinned foods should be in intact tins, with no bulges, rust marks or dents. Any damage may have allowed bacteria or other germs to enter the tin.

SEASONAL FRUITS AND VEGETABLES

Spring

apples (Bramley are the latest, available up to April/May)	lettuce oranges	spring greens

Summer

apricots	french beans	peas
asparagus	fresh herbs	radishes
beetroot	gooseberries	raspberries
blackberries	melons	rhubarb
blackcurrants	nectarines	runner beans
cherries	new potatoes	salad onions
cucumber	peaches	strawberries

Autumn

apples	curly kale	parsnips
blackberries	figs	pears
broccoli	grapes	plums
Brussels sprouts	kiwi fruits	potatoes
courgettes	late raspberries	spinach

Winter

apples	curly kale	onions
Brussels sprouts	Honeydew melons	parsnips
clementines	leeks	satsumas
		tangerines

BEST-BEFORE DATES

Pay attention to the 'best-before' and 'sell-by' dates. You can probably safely go a day after most of these dates, but remember that food is at its best when it is fresh. Every day past a sell-by date means a reduction in nutritional value. You may become ill if you eat meat and tinned goods that are too old (*see* p. 151).

FROZEN FOODS

Frozen foods should be at freezing temperature, and kept that way, to maintain their freshness and to ensure that they do not become contaminated. Choose packages from the bottom of the freezer (checking dates), and save your freezer shopping till last, so that you can get them home before they defrost.

EGGS, FISH AND MEAT

- Open egg cartons to inspect the eggs before you buy them, since cracked eggs are open to infection. If there is any 'fur' on the eggs, they may be mouldy. Hold the egg up to the light. The contents should be clear with a small air sac (less than 6mm deep). The yolk shouldn't move too much when the egg is turned.

- Raw meat should look firm, fresh and a healthy pink colour. Anything greying or bleached looking is not recommended for eating.

- Ensure that raw and cooked products do not come into contact with each other in the shop. Staff should be using different utensils to move them.

- Choose simple cuts of meat rather than products made with mixed meats, which are at greater risk of cross-contamination.

- Avoid ready-to-eat chickens which are one of the major causes of food poisoning in the UK.

- When choosing fish, don't buy anything that smells strongly.

- Don't freeze fresh fish: eat it the same day that it is purchased.

- When buying fresh, look for clear eyes, red gills, shiny skin and scales in place. The fish should feel firm and slightly resilient. Avoid fish with dull eyes or slimy skin.

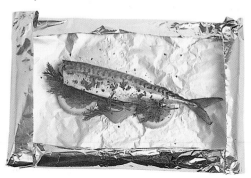

FOOD STORAGE

After choosing fresh produce, there are a number of things you can do to keep it healthy and nutritious until you are ready to eat it.

- The temperature of your refrigerator is one of the most important, and often under-rated safety points. If it is too cold, the food will partly freeze, causing damage. If it is too warm, the food may not be properly chilled, allowing bacteria to flourish. The temperature should be between 0° and 5°C. Defrost your fridge regularly to ensure it is functioning efficiently.

- Food should only be refrigerated for a short period of time. Milk lasts two to three days, meat shouldn't be kept for longer than 48 hours, poultry will last for 24 hours. Fresh fish should only be refrigerated for 12 hours after which it becomes a health hazard.

- Keep all fruits and vegetables, apart from potatoes and bananas, in the refrigerator if you have space.

- Make sure that all cooked foods are stored safely at the top of the refrigerator, and raw foods at the bottom where they can't drip on anything. Raw and cooked meats in particular should be kept completely separate in the refrigerator – in their own compartments, if possible.

- Remove fruits and vegetables from plastic bags to prevent moisture build up.

- Store potatoes in a paper bag in a dark place.

- Fruits that are left out to ripen in the sun should be
  eaten within a few days. Take note that bananas give
  off a gas that encourages other fruits and vegetables
  to ripen more quickly.

LEFTOVERS

- Leftovers should be kept for no longer than 24
  hours, and reheated only once, to piping hot.
  Anything left over after the second heating
  should be discarded.

- Never wrap fatty foods, such as cheese or meat,
  in cling film. Some of the chemicals in cling film
  react with fatty foods, and there is some
  evidence that they will impregnate the food. Put
  hot or fatty foods in a sealed airtight container, or
  in a bowl with clingfilm stretched across the top,
  but not touching the food.

- Never store uneaten food in tins or anything
  metallic. Transfer to a plastic container.

- Don't keep leftovers of custard, gravy or anything
  that has been made up from a powder containing
  meat, eggs, rice or dairy produce. These
  ingredients are most likely to harbour bacteria,
  which multiply when you add water and heat.

- Cool hot foods slightly before putting them in the
  refrigerator, to prevent raising the temperature of
  the fridge, which may encourage the build-up of
  moulds.

- Freezers and ice boxes of refrigerators are labelled with a star system and the labels on frozen food refer to this system when recommending the length of storage time.

- Keep your freezer temperature down to below –18°C. A full freezer helps you to do this, but purchase a freezer thermometer to check the temperature regularly.

HYGIENE IN THE KITCHEN

- Clean your refrigerator regularly with a diluted bleach solution, and mop up any spills immediately.

- Wash your hands before touching any food. Soap and warm water will be sufficient to kill the majority of germs, but take care to dry your hands afterwards on a clean, dry towel.

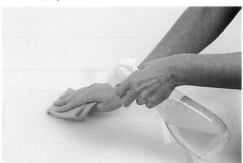

- Use one knife and chopping board for raw meat and seafood, and another for other foods, ensuring that they are washed carefully after each use.

- Wooden chopping boards are more germ-resistant than plastic ones, but should be washed carefully to clear away any bacteria that could be lurking.

- Don't wash your own dishes along with your pets' (unless you use a dishwasher, which washes at a high enough temperature to destroy bacteria). Similarly, ensure that all pets have their own dishes, and that they do not eat off yours.

HEALTHY COOKING

There are just a few simple rules for different categories of food:

Vegetables

- Wash salads carefully. Even ready-prepared salads may contain worms and other organisms, and may not have been washed adequately to get rid of any pesticide residues. There has even been a report of a woman finding a toad – alive – in her bag of ready-prepared salad!

- Scrubbing vegetables is better than peeling since many of the valuable vitamins and minerals are stored directly beneath their skins.

- Never soak vegetables for long periods. They are better washed briefly under running water so you don't allow the water-soluble vitamins (such as B and C) to leach out of them.

- Eat fresh fruits and vegetables raw whenever possible. Just five minutes of boiling reduces the thiamine (a B vitamin) content of peas by up to 40 percent. Similarly, boiling cabbage reduces its vitamin C content by up to 75 percent. Although vegetables are a good source of vitamin C, we often end up pouring most of it down the sink with the cooking water!

- Try to cook without water by steaming, stir-frying or briefly cooking in the microwave. To ensure optimal nutritional value, vegetables should be cooked for as short a time as possible.

- Roasting vegetables at a high temperature for a short period of time is a good way to ensure optimum nutritional content. Ensure they are still slightly crunchy when serving.

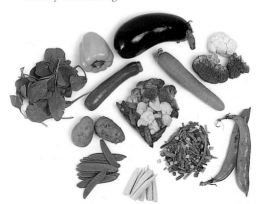

SAFE COOKING

- Cut off the fat from all types of meat, except organic. Fat is a notorious store for chemicals, including any growth enhancers given to the animals, or even pesticides used on their feed.

- Do not serve anything with raw or lightly cooked eggs to children, the elderly or anyone with an immune problem because of the risk of salmonella (*see* p. 151).

- Always use a clean teaspoon when tasting food while cooking.

- Thoroughly defrost all meat and cook-chilled meals before cooking, unless otherwise indicated on the package.

Meat

- Pork should always be cooked through to avoid the risk of food poisoning. Meat should reach a temperature of 70–75°c in the centre when it is done.

- Avoid deep-frying. Apart from the incredibly high fat content, this method of cooking destroys almost all the nutrients in the foods. If you must fry food, olive oil is probably the safest oil to use, but it should never be heated to smoking point.

- Grill food whenever possible. Grilling allows you to cook without the use of fat, and helps to maintain the nutritional content of the food.

- Browning vegetables and meats in a non-stick pan is a useful way of drawing out some of the fat in meat, and of changing the flavour of vegetables without allowing them to absorb unnecessary fat.

- Soups and casseroles are an excellent way to preserve nutritional content, as any vitamins and minerals lost in the cooking process will be found in the broth.

- Barbecued food can be unhealthy. Food tends to char on the outside, and remain undercooked on the inside, which can cause food poisoning.

Poultry

- Cook poultry in a slow oven until cooked through. Pierce it to see if the juices run clear. If they are still pink, cook for longer.

- Cook stuffing outside the poultry; when it is cooked inside, the bird may not cook thoroughly, and bacteria from the raw meat may survive.

Fish

- Lightly grill fish until it is tender but not raw.

- Poach fresh seafood gently, in as little water as possible.

Rice

- Rice should be cooked with the minimum of water, which is then absorbed into the rice and not discarded. If you have previously cooked vegetables, use the water to cook your rice, adding a little lemon juice to reduce starchiness.

What is in our food?

Nature supplies the planet with abundant varieties of food sources for the human body – fruits and fish, grains and meats – all of which are perfectly nutritious. But modern agriculture has upset the balance by applying chemical technology to farming. The majority of fruits and vegetables are sprayed with pesticides, grown on intensively farmed land, picked too early, artificially ripened, possibly waxed, and then sent halfway across the world to supermarkets.

Meat is no better! The growth of intensive farming of animals and the ever-increasing number of scares involving animal products is cause for concern.

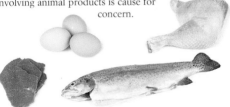

In the last decade the spotlight has focused on a number of food ingredients and additives, particularly those identified by E-numbers.

Don't panic, because considerable progress has been made towards understanding the risks, providing consumers with information and removing some of the most problematic additives.

FOOD ADDITIVES

A food additive is a substance added to food during its processing to preserve it or improve its colour, texture, flavour, or value. Here are some of the main types:

Flavourings Chemicals, used to intensify food flavours, such as monosodium glutamate (MSG or E621).

Sugar Sugars are an essential part of our diet, but too much can cause tooth decay (particularly in children) and contribute to obesity which, in turn, is linked to an increased risk of coronary heart disease and diabetes.

Super-sweeteners Modern sweeteners are used to add sweetness without the calories of sugar. They include saccharin and aspartame. Critics in the US allege that aspartame is responsible for a wide range of health problems.

Stimulants Caffeine is probably the most widely used legal stimulant. It is found in coffee, tea, many soft drinks and colas, headache tablets and other products. It excites the brain and even in low quantities it can cause headaches, digestive upsets, anxiety and depression.

Emulsifiers Used to stop mixtures (such as oils and vinegars in salad dressings) from separating.

Stabilizers Improve the texture of foods. Some natural stabilizers are still used, including lecithin.

Colouring Some food colourings have often been linked to health problems, and many manufacturers have begun to take note. Foods are now, on the whole, less vibrant in colour.

Preservatives Many foods go off fairly rapidly, particularly in hot weather, unless they are preserved in some way. Basic food preservatives include salt, vinegar and sugar, none of which is completely healthy. However, given that preservatives can prevent such potentially deadly diseases as botulism (*see* p. 151), they are clearly important in protecting our health.

Wax coatings Fruits are waxed to make them look shinier, and in some cases to protect them from going off quickly. The skins of some apples, lemons, melons, oranges and pineapples are waxed with animal products, of a sort. Shellac, an insect secretion, and beeswax are often used, which could prove unacceptable to some vegetarians.

E-NUMBERS

E-numbers are all substances that have been cleared for use as food additives in Europe and, officially, foods contain too little of them to do any harm. Some of them are healthy, such as E300, which is simply Vitamin C. Others are preservatives, which are necessary for the product to survive for any length of time.

The list of ingredients found on product labels gives the E-numbers contained in the product, but some manufacturers use the chemical name as well. Booklets listing the chemical names of E-numbers are available from big supermarkets.

READING THE LABELS

Food labelling is an important source of information for consumers about the composition of packaged foods. Government food, meat and poultry laws require a statement of ingredients on most food labels.

WHAT TO LOOK FOR

The main E numbers that have been linked with health problems of various descriptions include: E102, E110, E122, E123, E124, E127, E129, E131, E133, E142, E150C, E151, E153, E154, E155, E210-E224, E226, E227, E228, E232, E249, E250, E251, E252, E284, £285, E320, E321, E512, E533B, E621, E942, E954, E1440.

E310 to E312, E20 and E321 may be dangerous to asthmatics and to people who are sensitive to aspirin. They are also among the additives that are forbidden in baby foods.

E249 to E252 are nitrates, usually found in cured meats such as bacon. These additives can have harmful effects (*see* pp 96 and 154).

Healthy antioxidant E-numbers include those from E300 to 304 (Vitamin C) and E307 to 309 (Vitamin E).

The sweeter, more brightly coloured or flavoured a food, the higher the number of additives. Avoid these foods as far as possible.

Regulations require that ingredients be listed in order of predominance by their common, specific names.

The ingredients are listed by weight, so the first item on the list will be the one that makes up the majority of the contents. If you are buying a meat product, such as sausages, you'll want to see pork or beef in the number one position. Similarly, a fruit juice drink should have fruit listed first.

HIDDEN INGREDIENTS

Watch out for hidden ingredients. A product may not list 'sugar', for example, but sucrose, glucose, lactose, fructose and maltose are all sugars. Syrup and maltodextrin are also types of sugars, and should not appear in something claiming to be largely sugar-free.

USE-BY DATES

The main thing to check on the label is the 'use-by' date, which is the latest date at which the product can be guaranteed to be

INGREDIENTS

Sugar, Modified Starch, Whey Powder, Hydrogenated Vegetable Oil, Cream Powder, Dried Skimmed Milk, Milk Protein, Flavourings, Colours (Beta-carotene, Annatto)

NUTRITION INFORMATION

	Per 100g as packed	Per Serving
Energy	1670kJ/385kcal	410kJ/97kcal
Protein	4.1 g	1.0 g
Carbohydrate	74.0 g	18.5 g
- of which Sugars	54.0 g	13.5 g
Fat	8.2 g	2.1 g
- of which Saturates	7.2 g	1.8 g
Fibre	0.0 g	0.0 g
Sodium	0.3 g	0.1 g

safe to eat. The 'sell-by' date is one for shopkeepers, and you can normally eat the product up to three to four days after this date.

WHAT DO THE TERMS MEAN?

SUGAR

Sugar free: less than 0.5 grams (g) per serving

No added sugar, Without added sugar, No sugar added:
- No sugars added during processing or packing, including ingredients that contain sugars (for example, fruit juices, apple sauce, or dried fruit)

- Processing does not increase the sugar content above the amount naturally present in the ingredients.

- The food that it resembles and for which it substitutes normally contains added sugars

- If the food doesn't meet the requirements for a low- or reduced-calorie food, the product has a statement that the food is not low-calorie or calorie-reduced

Reduced sugar: at least 25 percent less sugar per serving than the normal product

FAT

Fat free: less than 0.5g of fat per serving

Saturated fat free: less than 0.5g per serving

Low fat: 3g or less per serving

Low saturated fat: 1g or less per serving and not more than 15 percent of calories from saturated fat

Reduced or Less fat: at least 25 percent less per serving than usual

Reduced or Less saturated fat: at least 25 percent less per serving than usual

CALORIES

Calorie free: fewer than 5 calories per serving

Low calorie: 40 calories or less per serving

Reduced or Fewer calories: at least 25 percent fewer calories per serving than usual

CHOLESTEROL

Cholesterol free: less than 2 milligrams (mg) of cholesterol and 2g or less of saturated fat per serving

Low cholesterol: 20mg or less and 2g or less of saturated fat per serving

Reduced or Less cholesterol: at least 25 percent less and 2g or less of saturated fat per serving than usual

SALT (SODIUM)

Sodium (salt) free: less than 5mg per serving

Low sodium (salt): 140mg or less per serving

Very low sodium (salt): 35mg or less per serving

Reduced or Less sodium (salt): at least 25 percent less per serving than usual

FIBRE

High fibre: 5g or more per serving. (Foods must meet the definition for low fat, or the level of total fat must appear next to the high-fibre claim.)

Good source of fibre: 2.5 g to 4.9 g per serving

More or Added fibre: at least 2.5 g more per serving than usual

NUTRITIONAL CONTENT

Nutritional content is also important. You should find information on the number of calories in the product, or in a percentage of the product, along with its carbohydrate, protein, fat, fibre and sodium content.

- **Carbohydrates** should be broken down into 'sugars' and 'others'. Sugars should form a smaller percentage of the carbohydrate total of a package.

- **Fat** is normally broken down into 'saturated' (unhealthy) and 'others'. Remember that your total fat intake for a day should be 30 percent of your total calorie intake: between 50 and 80 grams for most people.

EXPERTS RECOMMEND THE FOLLOWING GUIDELINE FOR YOUR FAT INTAKE:

If you eat this number of calories per day:	Total fat per day (grams)	Total saturated fat per day (grams)
1,600	53 or less	18 or less
2,000	65 or less	20 or less
2,200	73 or less	24 or less
2,500	80 or less	25 or less

So, if a takeaway sandwich listed 12g of fat, of which 8.8 were saturated, you would be consuming roughly a fifth of your fat intake for the day, and about a third of your saturated fat intake.

ON THE FARM

Recent food scares, and the growing concern about the welfare of animals, have caused the consumer to look more closely at how and where their food is produced.

ANTIBIOTICS

Animals raised in inadequate conditions suffer, not surprisingly, from stress, which lowers their immune function and they become more vulnerable to bacteria and viruses. To deal with this and other problems of over-crowding, the farming industry uses antibiotics to protect animals against disease and to make them grow faster. As a result, the vast majority of pigs and poultry are routinely given antibiotics in their feed or water.

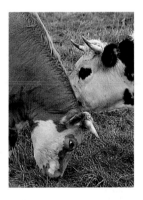

Worryingly, the over-use of antibiotics can lead to antibiotic resistance, which could mean that some of the antibiotics used in human medicine become less effective or even useless.

GROWTH HORMONES

The use of hormones to promote growth in food animals was banned in the EU in 1988, following consumer concerns about possible health effects.

BSE

Bovine spongiform encephalopathy (BSE) was probably caused by farmers feeding their cattle with contaminated animal proteins. The human variant, Creutzfeldt Jakob Disease (CJD), could be caught by people eating contaminated meat.

Regulations have now been passed to ensure that no more cattle feed is contaminated with animal proteins and the government and EU have declared that British beef is once again safe to eat. If you can afford it, you may prefer to buy organic meat, which has never been contaminated in this way (*see* p. 156).

SOMETHING FISHY?

Fish farming is generally more energy-efficient than rearing animals. In some ways it might seem to be at least part of the answer to the problems of over-fishing. Today, nearly 200 species of fish and shellfish are cultivated in ponds or coastal tanks and pens. Fish farming produces more than half of all the freshwater fish eaten around the world.

But industrial fish farming does have drawbacks. Feed for fish farms is often made from industrial fishing catches and contains chemicals designed to control

FOOD POISONING

This is an acute illness caused by eating food contaminated with harmful bacteria. Symptoms generally include vomiting and diarrhoea and appear within 12 to 24 hours after eating the food.

The **Salmonella** bacteria is found particularly in eggs and poultry. To avoid infection, wash your hands thoroughly after handling uncooked poultry, and don't eat raw or lightly cooked eggs. Most people recover within a few days but it can be dangerous for the young, the elderly, and anyone with an impaired immune system.

The **Listeria** bacteria can be found in certain soft cheeses, unpasteurized dairy products, and processed meat products such as pâtés. It can also harbour in pre-cooked foods, so ensure that they are heated right through. In pregnant women, listeriosis can damage the fetus.

E. coli infections have been hitting the headlines recently after serious outbreaks killed a number of people. It is imperative that you follow all the hygiene rules when handling meats and only buy mixed meat products such as sausages and meat pies from reputable sources.

Botulism is a rare but very serious form of food poisoning which is fatal in two-thirds of cases. It is found in improperly preserved foods such as tinned raw meats, but is destroyed by thorough cooking.

diseases and pests. Fish farms that are poorly sited or do not operate to high standards tend to have a higher incidence of disease, which therefore require treatment. Furthermore, the routine use of antibiotics in fish farming is causing concern, since it may lead to antibiotic resistance in humans!

WHICH FISH TO BUY

Your fishmonger will help you to choose fish that is farmed from a reputable, recognized organization. Organic fish is also available, though a little more expensive.

Fishing for tuna with long nets used to kill dolphins as well when they became entangled in the nets. These techniques have now been changed, but it is important only to buy tins of tuna labelled 'dolphin-friendly'.

CHICKEN AND EGGS

Chickens kept in battery farms are fed a wide range of chemicals to make them grow, and drugs to prevent the spread of disease in their often unhygienic conditions.

Free-range chicken is always best. If you can't afford it, look for 'corn-fed', or labels saying that the birds have been reared in 'humane' conditions.

Try to buy free-range eggs. If the cost is prohibitive, stick to free-range when you are eating the eggs alone (scrambled, or poached, for example),

WHAT DO THE LABELS MEAN?

'Free-range' eggs and poultry   Free-range tells you that far more space is required for the birds, which means better conditions.

'Organic'   Organic produce is strictly regulated and comes from animals kept under more natural conditions so they don't need drugs to prevent diseases caused by stress and overcrowding. They also live on drug-free, natural foods.

'Real meat'   Real meat suppliers put animal welfare first – also banning growth promoters and the use of drugs like antibiotics, unless the animal is genuinely in need of them.

and use ordinary supermarket eggs for cooking (making cakes or pancakes, for example).

FRUITS AND VEGETABLES

Fertilizers, pesticides and genetic engineering are topics of concern to the healthy eater.

FERTILIZERS

Intensive farming depletes the soil, creating a need for increasing amounts of fertilizer. This fertilizer eventually makes its way into our food through the plants we eat, and through the animals who ate the plants. Fertilizers are dangerous for a number of reasons:

- Fertilizers run into rivers – where the extra nutrients cause algae to grow faster and strip the water of oxygen, suffocating fish and other wildlife.

- Nitrates from nitrogen fertilizers gradually work their way down into underground water and contaminate the drinking water.

- Nitrates are also implicated in such human health problems as stomach cancer in adults and 'blue baby' syndrome in new-born infants.

PESTICIDES

- Pesticides are commonly sprayed to kill pests, but at the same time they contaminate the plants and the

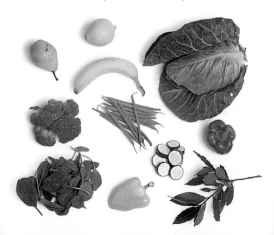

surrounding area, as well as the healthy animals and insects that would have eaten the pests in the natural order of things.

- Pesticides can damage our immune systems, making us more vulnerable to illness and disease. The immune systems of other animals are also affected.

- Much of the food that we eat contains measurable quantities of pesticide residues, even though the chemicals have been applied legally. Some imported foods may even contain residues of pesticides banned in the UK.

- Given that children are particularly vulnerable, and that we encourage them to eat lots of fruit and vegetables, their potential exposure is a matter of real concern.

GENETIC ENGINEERING

Genetic engineering, or modification, involves removing genetic material (genes) from one species, and implanting it in another, to create 'improved' versions. It began with the Flavr Savr tomato, which was implanted with a gene to prevent it from ripening too quickly, and ultimately rotting. Fruit such as avocados, bananas, cantaloupe and chantelais melons, strawberries and tomatoes have all now been experimentally engineered to slow rotting – and to retain taste.

In another process, the pectin levels of tomatoes have been altered by genetic engineering, to produce denser fruit for use in tomato purée. This makes a thicker paste – and uses less energy for processing.

There are also plants that have had their genes modified to resist different insecticides, for example, and animals have had their genes altered to produce 'better' breeds.

Should we be worried? The answer is yes. Genetic modification is, to many people, a dangerous game. Still a relatively new concept, there is not enough research to show what the real dangers may be.

And, our health may be at risk: new proteins in food products resulting from genetic engineering may be capable of triggering food allergies. Genetic engineering could result in food which looks both tasty and nutritious, but does not provide the nutrients we need.

GOING ORGANIC

Organic food is more than just a new trend in eating – it is the food of the future, and one of the few ways to eat safely, and to be sure that what you are eating is healthy.

WHY ORGANIC FOOD IS BETTER

Organic fruits and vegetables are grown without artificial fertilizers or pesticides, in ground that is tested and declared free of any contamination.

- Nothing that is labelled organic has been genetically modified (*see* p. 155).
- Organically raised animals are given comfortable surroundings, and fed organically produced food.
- Land used for grazing must not have pesticides or chemicals sprayed on it.

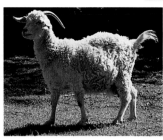

- No antibiotics or other drugs are given to organically raised animals, unless they are genuinely ill.

- Animals are not fed anything containing animal products, if they are natural herbivores (like cows), and most of their food is found in their natural environment – the fields of the farm.

- Organic animals were safe from the BSE scandal, because they were fed on natural foods. No BSE has been found in cattle born on organic farms that had been certified organic before 1985.

- Organic food tastes better!

ARE THERE ANY DRAWBACKS?

Although the price is coming down, organic food is still more expensive than other produce. It can also be difficult to find a wide variety of products, although that, too, is improving.

BUYING ORGANIC FOOD

Most supermarkets have responded to consumer demand and are now stocking ever-increasing supplies of organic food. Demand has meant that the price differential between organic and conventionally farmed produce is decreasing, and will continue to do so.

Why is it more expensive?

The cost of farming organically is higher than conventional farming because its producers do not receive the same subsidies that support intensive farming, and because it's cheaper to keep animals indoors in crowded conditions.

Appearance

The appearance of organic food can sometimes be off-putting: organic fruits, for instance, are not waxed and may look less shiny, and less colourful than their conventionally grown cousins. Nutritionally, however, the organic fruit wins hands down. Remember that in nature, nothing is perfect. Imperfect-looking produce is

---

THE SOIL ASSOCIATION

The Soil Association campaigns on organic issues, provides certification and offers advice to farmers on converting to organic cultivation and farming methods. Look for the 'Soil Association' logo on organic foods. The best way of tracking down local companies are through the essential guides *Where to Buy Organic Food*, compiled by the Soil Association, or *The Organic Directory*, published by Green Earth Books.

not nutritionally or in any other way substandard. We have to re-educate ourselves to walk past the 'perfect' produce and choose products that are better for us, for our children and for our environment.

Organic priorities

If you can't afford to eat all organic, choose meat, eggs and root vegetables first and foremost. These are the products most likely to contain dangerous chemicals as a result of intensive farming.

Children are most at risk of chemical residues and should be given organic food whenever possible. The elderly, and anyone with a weakened immune system, should also consider eating organic as a priority.

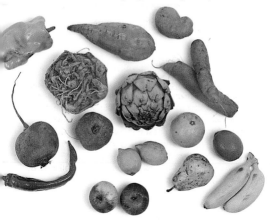

Healthy drinking

What we drink is just as important as the food we choose to eat. Good drinking habits will enhance a healthy diet, and help to make up for a poor one.

WATER

Water is essential to life. Without water we cannot survive for more than a few days, whereas we could live for several weeks without food. In the West, we take a clean water supply for granted, and water is the mainstay of the majority of drinks we consume throughout the day.

Fresh, clean water plays an important role in our bodies. It is crucial to the digestion of food and the absorption of nutrients. If you don't drink enough water between meals, your mouth becomes slow to produce saliva and digestion suffers. Water also eliminates wastes from our bodies.

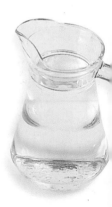

Experts recommend that we drink at least 8–10 glasses of fresh, pure water each day to cleanse our bodies and provide it with the raw material it needs to survive.

Water on Tap

In the UK, our water supply is reliable and clean. In fact, it is constantly checked for accidental contamination that may occur from industrial effluents, and agricultural run-offs. The material used to make the pipes is also checked for safety. Chemicals are added to our water to ensure that it is clean and pure, including chlorine, ferric sulphate and lime, and these levels are carefully controlled.

But even purified water can contain traces of potentially harmful substances, such as oestrogens. Lead can seep into it from household pipes; small quantities of nitrates can be found in it; and experts believe that the fluoride added to water in some areas can cause teeth to mottle and bones to become brittle.

Although in theory tap water should be safe to drink, if we increase our water intake substantially – to about 10 glasses a day, as recommended – the associated risks necessarily increase.

Filtering

One answer is to filter your water. A kitchen water filter reduces your chances of drinking unwanted metals and chemical residues. Choose a filter than removes pesticides, chlorine, lead and copper. There are many types of filters, some of which can be plumbed into your kitchen sink, but even a simple filter will do a great deal towards cutting out chemicals and improving the taste of the water.

HEALTHY WATER

- Filtered water is probably best, unless there is something wrong with your mains water.

- Change the filters as often as the manufacturer recommends and let the cold tap run for 30 seconds before using the water.

- Buy bottled water if you prefer the taste.

- Don't drink bottled water past its best-before date.

- Drink still bottled water rather than sparkling.

- Look for brands that are low in sodium.

- Drink 8 to 10 glasses of water a day!

BOTTLED WATER

There are many different kinds of bottled water, some from wells, some from natural springs, and some from ordinary tap water that has been reprocessed. They may be still, naturally carbonated or artificially carbonated. Some contain considerable amounts of dissolved minerals, which may be naturally present, or added later. Others may have a low mineral content.

Benefits of bottled water

- Bottled water can be a good source of minerals. People with trace mineral deficiencies report feeling better when they change to a mineral-rich water.

- Because bottlers must protect their reputations, springs are often guaranteed to be free of pesticide residues and other contaminants. Bottled waters are also much more likely to be free of, or lower in nitrates.

Drawbacks of bottled water

- Some brands have been found to contain more bacteria than tap water. By law, bacterial content is checked when the water is bottled, but if it sits in a bottle for several months, the content is bound to increase. Sparkling water is safer than still in this respect, since the 'fizz' of the carbon dioxide helps to prevent the multiplication of bacteria.

- But too much sparkling water can damage teeth, because carbon dioxide in water forms an acid.

- Some bottled waters contain a lot of sodium (salt) which can be dangerous for babies and children and anyone with high blood pressure. Look for brands that contain less than 20 mg sodium per litre.

- Fizzy mineral water 'with a hint of' fruit juice tends to be artifically sweetened and flavoured.

- It can be expensive if it's your main source of drinking water.

COFFEE OR TEA?

Coffee and tea contain caffeine, which is a drug. It stimulates the brain, and is also a diuretic, which means that it stimulates the flow of urine. Caffeine gives a burst of energy when you drink it, but shortly afterwards, you experience a slump, which is why so many people go back for another cup.

IS COFFEE GOOD FOR YOU?

- Coffee is processed with an amazing array of chemicals and there are lots of pesticides and other chemicals used to grow it. Switch to organic coffee if you can afford it.

- Coffee also contains a great deal of caffeine – the stronger the coffee, the more caffeine it contains.

- If you drink more than eight cups of coffee a day, you can experience irregular heartbeat, confusion, ringing in the ears, stomach upsets and even convulsions.

- Both tea and coffee reduce the absorption of iron and zinc. Try to avoid drinking coffee with meals, or with any supplements you are taking.

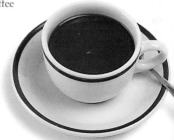

- Decaffeinated coffee may be lower in caffeine, but it is not any better for you. Indeed, the process of decaffeinating actually increases the chemical content. Why not try one of the natural, healthy alternatives to coffee: dandelion root coffee is a good option, and has the added benefit of cleansing the liver.

- If you do drink coffee, make sure you drink plenty of fresh, filtered or bottled water to help cleanse your system.

WHAT ABOUT TEA?

Tea is a slightly different story. Tea does have some health-giving properties, and as long as you don't drink it too strong, should only have about 60 per cent of the caffeine in coffee. It also contains 'tannins', which are believed to help prevent some forms of heart disease. Tea also contains flavonoids, which are 'antioxidant' (*see* p. 49). Green tea is believed to improve resistance to stomach and skin cancers, and stimulates the immune system.

Herbal teas and tisanes

The healthy properties of herbal teas and tisanes are well known. They cleanse and strengthen the body, and have a wide range of therapeutic benefits. They do not normally contain any caffeine. Drink them sweetened with a little honey, or freshened with a slice of lemon.

Here are some of the best teas to try for various ailments:

- **For calming the nerves, inducing sleep**: chamomile, limeflower, passion flower, red clover
- **For infections or colds**: rosehip, comfrey, aniseed, licorice, sage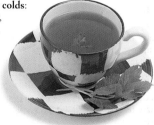
- **Indigestion or tummy ache**: peppermint, dill, fennel, lemongrass, aniseed, lemon balm
- **As a tonic**: Nettle, mint, ginseng, rosemary, raspberry and strawberry leaf. Caution: pregnant women should not drink raspberry leaf tea.
- **Diuretics for weight loss and the kidneys**: celery seed, dandelion, couchgrass, golden rod, agrimony

You can also drink herbal teas for their flavour alone. Delicious blends are now available from most supermarkets and healthfood shops.

ALCOHOL

Alcohol is one of the more popular social drinks, and regular intake has become both a part of our culture and our daily life. It's no longer considered 'taboo' to drink alone. Alcohol problems in women are on the increase: more than 520,000 women in the UK now drink more than 35 units a week, and half of those drink up to 8 units daily (about a bottle of wine).

WHY IS IT BAD?

People who regularly drink a bottle of wine, or its equivalent, in the course of a day will be open to liver damage, nutritional deficiency (alcohol robs the body of B vitamins in particular), brain shrinkage and a host of other conditions, including digestive problems and impaired memory. Fertility is also affected by drinking, because alcohol affects the hormones. Women drinking three or more drinks a day have an increased risk of breast cancer.

WHAT ARE THE EFFECTS?

- The effects of alcohol on the human body depend on the amount of alcohol in the blood. This varies according to the rate at which you drink, the rate at which your system absorbs and metabolizes alcohol, and your body weight.

- Studies indicate that women's stomachs contain relatively smaller amounts of an enzyme that breaks down alcohol than men, so relatively more alcohol enters the bloodstreams of women when drinking.

- One or two drinks can cause a feeling of relaxation and a mild sensation of euphoria. Shy people may feel more confident, and many people find it easier to socialize after one or two drinks.

SAFE DRINKING

- **Set a limit** If you know how much you are going to drink before you take your first sip, it will be easier to stick to that limit, even if you are pressured by friends to have more.

- **Make it last** If you drink slowly, you'll give your liver a chance to metabolize the alcohol so it won't build up in your body. Make each drink last more than half an hour.

- **Eat with your drink** Eating will slow down the rate at which alcohol is absorbed, but avoid salty foods such as peanuts that will make you thirsty and tempt you to drink more.

- **Dilute your drink** Start with a regular measure, but when it's half gone, add water or soda. Each time your glass is half empty, add more water.

- **Drink water** If you're thirsty, your body wants water not alcohol. If you drink a big glass of water first, you are more likely to drink alcohol in moderation.

- **Don't binge** Drinking seven units on Friday night, and seven more on Saturday can dramatically increase your blood pressure and your potential for blood clots.

- **Call a cab** Alcohol is involved in nearly half of all fatal automobile accidents.

- However, after three or four drinks, we will experience reduced co-ordination, hampered speech, slow reaction time, decreased inhibitions, and impaired judgement. Five or more drinks generally cause noticeable co-ordination and speech difficulties, inappropriate emotional reactions, drowsiness, and abusive or aggressive behaviour.

NOT ALL DOOM AND GLOOM

If you rarely overindulge, but you do sip a glass of wine at the end of the day, chances are you will live longer, and experience a better quality of life. One or two units of alcohol a day helps to relieve stress, helps you to think more clearly, to fend off heart disease and promotes longevity.

Eric Rimm, a nutritional epidemiologist at the Harvard University School of Public Health in Boston, says: 'If someone can control her alcohol consumption, then a glass of wine, a can of beer or a mixed drink a day can extend her life. In fact, death rates for people who savour a drink a day are 16 percent lower than for people who either drink more or nothing at all.'

THE UNIT SYSTEM

One unit is a half-pint of average strength beer (about 4 percent), or a single of 70 proof spirit, or one glass of wine or sherry. Experts recommend that women drink no more than 14 units a week, and men no more than 21.

SOFT DRINKS

Water is always the best drink when you are thirsty, but there are other options, some of which are very nutritious. We'll look at the healthy options first.

Fresh fruit and vegetable juices

- A glass of fresh fruit juice is considered to be the equivalent of a serving of fresh fruit, and will contain at least the recommended daily intake of vitamin C. In fact, fresh fruit and vegetable juices are essential parts of anti-cancer diets.

- Raw juices do most of the things that solid raw foods do, but in a way that places minimum strain on the digestive system. The concentrated vitamins, minerals, trace elements, enzymes, sugars and proteins they contain are absorbed into the bloodstream almost as soon as they reach the stomach and small intestine.

- If you are worried that you are eating insufficient fresh vegetable and fruit servings throughout the week, consider purchasing a juicer and making your own fresh juices regularly. Mix fruits and vegetables together for delicious taste combinations. Fresh fruit juices should be poured on to ice as soon as they are prepared, to reduce oxidation. Sealed, they can be kept in the refrigerator for several hours.

- Fresh fruit and vegetable juices are also high in fibre, and may need to be diluted for children, to avoid runny bowel movements. They are also high in natural, 'healthy' sugars, but care should be taken not to drink too much between meals, when sugars can damage your teeth.

NEXT BEST ...

Next best are freshly squeezed juices available from the supermarket. Remember, however, that they begin to lose their nutritional value from the moment they are opened. You are better off buying small cartons and finishing them within a few hours.

Juices made from concentrates tend to be much higher in sugar, and lower in vitamins and minerals. They are, however, much more nutritious than squashes and fizzy drinks, and are best drunk diluted with fresh water.

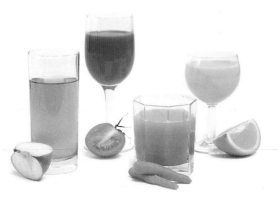

FIZZY DRINKS

The majority of fizzy drinks contain nothing but artificial sweeteners, flavours, sugar, caffeine and water. Some fizzy drinks may contain a little fruit juice, but not normally enough to make them worth buying. The best advice is to avoid them.

What are the problems?

- First of all, most fizzy drinks do not contain any nutrition. Many people fill up on them, leaving no room for more nutritious options.

- Fizzy drinks usually contain sugar. A 330ml (12oz) can (almost 2 glasses) of a fizzy drink, such as cola, contains the equivalent of 7 tsp of sugar!

- The 'fizz' in fizzy drinks contains an acid which can rot teeth. Add that to the amount of sugar that is in most fizzy drinks, and you have the perfect recipe for tooth decay.

- Sugar-free or artificially sweetened brands are not healthier. While they don't have the sugar and calories of regular soft drinks, they simply replace one bad thing (sugar) with another (artificial sugar). And as bad as sugar is, it's still better for you than artificial sweeteners, says the US Center for Science in the Public Interest. At least two artificial sweeteners – acesulfame-K and saccharin – may promote cancer, according to a new study.

- High quantities of fizzy drinks can affect the health of your digestive system. In some parts of the country, children suffer from the oral equivalent of Crohn's disease, with mouth ulcers, bleeding and pain.

SQUASHES

Squashes have always been popular, because they are cheap and you can dilute them fairly heavily. Squashes are, however, mainly sugar syrups, and even reduced-sugar brands are high in calories and very bad for dental health. Highly sweetened drinks actually increase the body's need for water, so they are not the best option for quenching thirst. There are many varieties of fruit squash, including high-juice fruit squash.

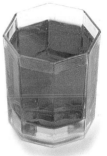

Watch out for 'sugar-reduced' brands. These often contain artificial sweeteners, which can be unhealthy (*see* p. 142).

HEALTHY TEETH

The following plan can help to prevent tooth decay.

- Juices must be diluted for between-meal drinks. Water is always the best drink between meals.

- Don't eat sweets, especially between meals. If you do want a sweet treat, eat it after your main meal, when the saliva produced from eating will reduce the damage.

- Eat chewy (but not sweetened) foods, such as raw fruit and vegetables, for gum health.

- Ensure a balanced diet during pregnancy to strengthen the teeth of an unborn child.

- Brush your teeth at least twice a day, after meals. Ask your dentist to show you the correct way to brush, and use a plaque-disclosing tablet every few weeks to highlight the areas you miss. Use dental floss carefully to avoid gum damage.

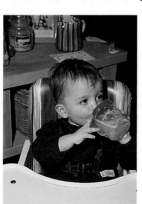

- Fluoride can be given to children under 12 to help strengthen teeth, but watch out for excess fluoride which can cause mottling of the teeth. If your water is fluoridated, you do not need extra fluoride.

- Remember that toothpaste contains fluoride. Only a pea-sized drop of toothpaste should be used for cleaning children's teeth.

Food for health

Foods not only build our body and provide us with the energy to undertake bodily functions, but they can affect our emotions, health and behaviour. Research indicates that a poor diet – one that is unbalanced, excessive or inadequate – may be a leading cause of illness in the Western world.

SPECIAL DIETS

Changing your diet can make an enormous difference in the way you look and feel, and can improve your health dramatically. Here are some practical tips for dealing with common health problems.

ANAEMIA

Avoid: foods and drinks that inhibit iron absorption, such as coffee, tea, alcohol, wheat bran; or those processes which cause vitamin loss (vitamins B and C), such as incorrect storage, long cooking times.
Eat: mineral- and vitamin-rich organ meats once or twice a week (but not if pregnant or planning a pregnancy; see your doctor), along with fish and/or vegetable proteins (pulses, nuts, seeds). Include plenty of green leafy vegetables and dried fruit such as apricots and figs, which are high in iron. Seeds are high in iron, and a good source of polyunsaturated fatty acids.

ARTHRITIS

Avoid: dairy foods, saturated fat, salty or pickled foods, food additives, acid fruit (e.g. berries, and citrus fruit), fried foods, tea, coffee, sugar, soft drinks and spirits, all of which place strain on the system. There is some evidence that chronic arthritis might be related to food intolerance, and eliminating possible suspects will help. Reduce intake of potatoes, tomatoes, bell peppers and aubergines – the nightshade family of vegetables – which can exacerbate arthritis and rheumatism.

Eat: a mainly vegetarian diet with a little oily fish two or three times a week. Meat and saturated fat can exacerbate the condition, while oily fish is high in essential fatty acids, which are preventative. Increase intake of anti-oxidant vegetables and fruit. Increase intake of raw and lightly cooked vegetables, which help to cleanse the blood. Drink vegetable juices instead of fruit juice, which is fairly acidic.

ASTHMA

Avoid: common allergens e.g. citrus. Animal proteins can exacerbate the condition.
Eat: plenty of freshly ground mixed seeds, especially pumpkin seeds, which are high in vitamins, minerals and essential fatty acids. Eat mainly vegetable protein such as tofu, seed vegetables and beans. Drink plenty of diluted fruit juices and bottled or filtered water, between meals. Drink a small amount of diluted cider vinegar with the main meal of the day for its antispasmodic properties.

CANDIDIASIS AND THRUSH

Avoid: all sugar (and sweet fruit, initially), refined foods, alcohol, tea, coffee, smoked/pickled meat or fish and fermented foods, which 'feed' the candida. Reduce the amount of meat and dairy foods, which can cause mucus to build up.
Eat: raw vegetables, which boost the immune system and are full of nutrients. Increase vegetables and fruit high in vitamins A and C, and antioxidants to keep the immune system active. Drink three to four glasses of cranberry juice a day, which helps to prevent secondary infection.

CYSTITIS AND URINARY TRACT INFECTIONS

Avoid: red meat, which can exacerbate the condition. Reduce intake of dairy foods, especially milk, which can encourage the build-up of mucus and bacteria.
Eat: more antioxidant fruit and vegetables to boost immunity. Eat mainly plant protein, with a little oily fish,

poultry, and lean meat. Drink cranberry juice in between meals (helps to remove *E. coli* – often the cause of urinary tract infections – from the bladder wall). Increase level of fluid intake to around two litres a day, between meals to flush the system.

Depression

Avoid: refined foods, foods containing additives (especially colours, preservatives, and artificial sweeteners), sugar, alcohol, tea, coffee, colas, cheese, and red wine (and other tyramine-containing foods), drugs (other than those prescribed by your physician). All of these things can exacerbate depression and anxiety.

Eat: fruit as the only source of sugar to prevent blood sugar swings. Increase intake of raw and lightly cooked vegetables. Increase intake of freshly ground mixed seeds, including linseeds for their essential fatty acids. Eat organic produce

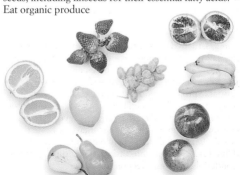

whenever possible, to avoid toxins that might
overwhelm your system, or to which you may be allergic.

DIGESTIVE PROBLEMS

Avoid: refined foods, sugar, alcohol and caffeine, which
can be hard on the digestive system. Avoid mixing
concentrated starches and concentrated proteins in the
same meal, which can impair the digestive process.
Eat: Jerusalem artichokes – they act as a digestive, and
encourage the liver to produce bile. Increase intake of
fibrous vegetables, and rice and barley bran (as
wholegrain) to encourage the digestive action. Increase
intake of antioxidant vegetables and fruit. Eat live
yoghurt daily (if allergic to dairy milk, use live soya
yoghurt) to encourage the growth of healthy bacteria
(flora). Increase intake of water and other fluids in
between meals. Increase intake of cellulose and pectin
fibres (omit wheat fibre) for regularity.

ECZEMA

Avoid: saturated fat, hydrogenated fat, refined foods,
food additives, common food allergens and alcohol, all
of which can exacerbate the problem.
Eat: oily fish (herring, mackerel and salmon) and
vegetable protein (soya) instead of meat, poultry and
dairy proteins. The essential fatty acids help the immune
system, preventing allergic reactions, as well as
encouraging skin health. Increase intake of freshly
ground mixed seeds, especially pumpkin seeds. Sip
diluted cider vinegar with main meal of the day. It has a
wonderful cleansing effect on the body.

HAEMORRHOIDS AND VARICOSE VEINS

Avoid: or reduce the amount of animal produce (meat and dairy products), which are hard on the circulatory system.

Eat: some whole linseeds with your daily mixed seeds; take a full glass of water with these. These help the circulatory system and promote the health of your veins. Increase the amount of antioxidant-containing vegetables.

HEART DISEASE AND CIRCULATORY PROBLEMS

Avoid: salt, coffee, sugar, refined grains, hydrogenated fats, fried foods, fatty or processed meats, full fat milk and cheese, cream – all of which contain saturated fats that can cause heart disease. Reduce intake of alcohol (maximum two units, preferably red wine, once or twice a week).

Eat: predominantly vegetable protein, such as soybeans, tofu, beans, with oily fish taken two or three times a week. Increase foods for nourishment of blood vessels, such as dark green and orange vegetables, peas, oats

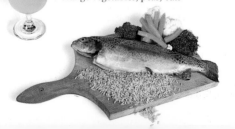

onions, garlic, fresh wheatgerm, sunflower seeds, sprouted seeds, lecithin, freshly ground linseeds.

IRRITABLE BOWEL SYNDROME

Avoid: alcohol, coffee, strong spices, refined foods and sugar, food additives, milk, and other common allergens.
Eat: lots of antioxidant vegetables and fruit, which can help the healing process. Increase intake of water and other fluids in between meals to encourage digestive action and prevent constipation. Water will also soothe inflamed membranes. Increase intake of cellulose and pectin fibres (omit wheat fibre) for regularity.

MENSTRUAL DISORDERS

Avoid: refined foods, coffee, salt, sugar and alcohol which can exacerbate the problems.
Eat: five or six small meals a day, having a small amount of protein to balance the carbohydrate at each meal. This will prevent blood sugar swings. Balance animal proteins (oily fish and lean meat) with vegetable proteins (seeds, nuts, soya, pulses and seed vegetables). Increase intake of a wide range of fruit and vegetables, especially dark green vegetables. Increase intake of freshly ground mixed seeds, especially sesame and pumpkin, for their essential fatty acids.

ME (MYALGIC ENCEPHALOMYELITIS)

Avoid: all stimulants (tea, coffee, alcohol, colas), 'rich food', refined food and sugar, which are hard on the system. Reduce foods that are difficult to digest (meat,

dairy, some grains and pulses).
Eat: tofu, millet, quinoa, 'seed' vegetables, seeds and
some nuts, and fish. Increase intake of antioxidant
nutrients. Eat freshly ground mixed seeds for their
essential fatty acids. Increase intake of lightly steamed
vegetables, which can help boost the immune system.

OSTEOPOROSIS

Avoid: animal protein (except fish and yoghurt), coffee,
alcohol, refined carbohydrates and sweets, which can
encourage bone loss. Reduce intake of refined
carbohydrate and sweet food (encourages alkalinity of
digestive juices and renders calcium insoluble).
Eat: freshly ground mixed seeds, especially sesame and
pumpkin for their essential fatty acids. Increase intake of
vegetables and fruit for their nutritional value.

PRE-MENSTRUAL SYNDROME (PMS)

Avoid: or reduce intake of red meat, and alcohol, which
can exacerbate the problem.
Eat: five or six small meals a day and include a little
protein with each one to prevent blood sugar swings.
Increase intake of a wide range of fruit and vegetables,
especially dark green vegetables, for B-vitamins and
antioxidants. Eat at least some raw vegetables and
sprouted seeds and beans daily – this will also increase
your daily fibre intake. Increase intake of freshly ground
mixed seeds (sunflower, sesame, pumpkin and linseed)
for essential fatty acids. Drink bottled or filtered water
between meals (to avoid oestrogens in tap water, and to
help prevent water retention).

PSORIASIS

Avoid citrus fruit, tomatoes, red meat, saturated fats, hydrogenated fats, sweets, alcohol and refined carbohydrates, all of which can exacerbate the condition.

Eat: at least some raw vegetables daily for their nutritional content, and to cleanse the blood. Increase intake of freshly ground mixed seeds, especially pumpkin seeds, for their essential fatty acids. Increase intake of vegetable fibre and pectin (apples, carrots) to aid elimination.

SINUSITIS

Eat: lots of dark green vegetables (some raw) and fruit. Increase intake of onions and garlic (steamed onions are very beneficial) to reduce catarrh, and for their anti-bacterial action.

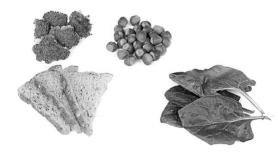

STRESS AND INSOMNIA

Avoid: refined and processed foods, caffeine-containing beverages (tea, coffee, colas), food additives, overcooked food, table salt, alcohol, which can stimulate the system.
Eat: extra wheatgerm or oatgerm added to cereals, for their B-vitamins. Drink chamomile or passion flower teas for their soothing effect. Eat ground mixed seeds, especially sesame (or use sesame oil in salads), for their high levels of zinc, which can help sleep.

ALLERGIES AND INTOLERANCE

Food allergies and intolerances (milder forms of allergy) are particularly difficult to pinpoint as a cause of illness, and many of us may be intolerant without knowing it. If you crave certain foods, and these foods form a major part of your daily diet, you may well be intolerant.

People who have had difficulty shifting weight, or who suffer from overwhelming fatigue, sleep disturbances, dry skin or food cravings often experience a complete alleviation of symptoms when they remove certain foods from their daily diets. In most cases, excess weight, bloating and fatigue disappear, and they feel much healthier overall. This doesn't mean that suspect foods need to be avoided for ever – they should be eaten as 'treats', rather than used as staples of the diet, and they should be avoided when you are feeling rundown, tired, bloated or depressed.

WHAT CAN YOU DO?

- Anyone who suffers from eczema, asthma, dermatitis, migraine, fatigue, depression, aching muscles, mouth ulcers, water retention, wind, nausea, Crohn's disease, irritable bowel syndrome or constipation, should consider the possibility that food may be the cause.

- You can carry out an exclusion test at home if you are concerned about a certain food. It is important to maintain a balanced diet, so very strict elimination or exclusion diets should only be carried out under reputable professional supervision. Keep a food diary throughout a period of exclusion so that you can look back at your patterns of eating and symptoms. Introduce foods in small quantities, one at a time, to see if you get any kind of a reaction before having normal helpings again.

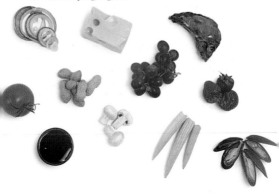

Glossary

acidophilus This is one of the main types of 'friendly' bacteria that lives in our digestive systems. It helps to prevent 'unfriendly' bacteria from multiplying, forms part of our immune defence system, helps our bowel function and produces vitamins and other substances. It is found in live yoghurt.

allergen Something that causes an allergy in susceptible people. For example, gluten would be an allergen for people who are sensitive to wheat.

antidiabetic Something that works to reduce or prevent the symptoms of diabetes, such as low blood sugar levels.

antigen A substance, which is usually foreign to the body, that causes the immune system to form antibodies in response.

atrio-ventricular This refers to the four chambers of the heart.

calcification The hardening of tissues, such as bones, when there is an excess of calcium,

and they become impregnated by calcium build-ups.

candida A condition in which a type of yeast – candida albicans – proliferates in the body. An over-growth of candida in the intestines is known as candidiasis; when it over-grows in the mouth or vagina, it is called 'thrush'.

cell respiration The 'breathing' action of cells as they exchange gases and other substances with other cells.

cellulose An important dietary fibre that is a constituent of the walls of plant cells. It is not digestible by humans, which makes it a good 'cleansing' substance, as it passes through our digestive system.

co-factor A helper, or a substance that is important in the process described.

detoxify When toxins build up in the body, they need to be excreted. When you detoxify, you cleanse the body of toxins. The liver is often the site of built-up toxins, and there are many diets available to detoxify the liver.

dilation When something dilates, or expands.

endocrine system The glands that secrete hormones into the bloodstream. It includes the thyroid, pituitary and adrenal glands.

enzyme An enzyme is a protein produced by the body that helps the metabolism to function. The best known enzymes are digestive enzymes, which break down food, allowing it to be absorbed by the body.

essential amino acid Amino acids are needed to make all the components of the body, including enzymes, blood, hormones, antibodies, hair, skin, bones and tissues. Essential amino acids are those that the body is incapable of making itself and which must be obtained from the diet.

fats (monounsaturated and polyunsaturated) These generally derive from plants and are liquid at room temperature. The difference between them is the way the molecules are bonded together. Olive oil is a monounsaturated fat, while corn oil is polyunsaturated.

fats (saturated and unsaturated) Saturated fats are generally of animal origin and are solid at room temperature. They are more likely to clog the arteries, causing heart disease. Unsaturated fats are of plant origin and are liquid at room temperature.

heavy metals These are metals, such as mercury and lead, which the body finds very difficult to excrete. When they build up, they can cause illness.

histamine This is a substance released by the body in response to an allergen. The effects of histamine include dilated capillaries, reduced blood pressure and increased stomach acid production, skin redness, swelling, or constriction of the breathing passages.

hormone A substance which regulates the activity of an organ or a group of cells. For example, adrenaline is a hormone that is released by the adrenal glands.

hydrogenation This is a process used by food manufacturers to make a liquid a solid. For example, corn oil may be hydrogenated to make a corn oil margarine. The process involves lots of chemicals, and is not considered to be very healthy.

hyperglycaemia and hypoglycaemia Hyperglycaemia is high blood sugar; hypoglycaemia is low blood sugar.

inorganic compounds Something that is not living, or derived from something that is living. A mineral is an inorganic compound.

insulin This is a hormone produced by the pancreas, which is involved in the control of our blood sugar levels.

iu An international unit, used to measure the fat soluble vitamins, such as A, D and E. For example, the iu of Vitamin A is 0.3 micrograms.

mcg Micrograms, a unit of measurement equivalent to 10^{-6} (one millionth) of a gram.

metabolism All the processes that take place in our bodies that result in growth, energy production, waste elimination and many other functions.

miso A Japanese food made from soya beans (and sometimes grains such as rice or barley) and sea salt fermented for 3 years. It is said to be excellent for people with weak digestive systems, and for those who have been taking antibiotics, to help increase the population of 'healthy' bacteria (*see* **acidophilus**).

monosaccharide Simple carbohydrates, or sugars. They are the least complex carbohydrates, which means that they are most easily digested (not always a good thing in the case of carbohydrates). They can cause surges and then drops in energy.

nutrient A part of our diet that is essential to our life and health. They are classified as macronutrients (carbohydrates, fat, protein, dietary fibre, and in some cases essential fatty acids) and micronutrients (vitamins, minerals and trace elements).

oestrogens The hormones which promote female characteristics and reproductive functions. They include oestradiol, oestrone and oestriol.

osteoporosis A disease in which the bones become extremely porous, fracture easily, and heal slowly. This most often occurs in women following menopause and can lead to curvature of the spine from vertebral collapse.

polysaccharide A complex carbohydrate, which is less easily absorbed or digested by the body, making it a good source of long-term energy.

precursor A biochemical substance, usually in a chain of reactions, that is essential for the creation of a more stable or definitive product. For example, betacarotene is a precursor of vitamin A, which means that it is a substance necessary for it to be absorbed and utilized in our bodies.

renal Related to the kidneys. For example, renal function is the function of the kidneys.

saccharide A simple sugar that is a type of carbohydrate.

tempeh A fermented soya product which originated in the Far East, and has a firm texture, suitable for slicing. Tempeh is often used as a meat substitute by vegetarians.

tofu Soya milk curd pressed into blocks. It is rich in protein and highly versatile for use in cooking. It is often used as a meat substitute by vegetarians.

toxoplasmosis A disease caused by *Toxoplasma gondii*, which is frequently carried by cats. It causes fever, swollen lymph nodes, and lesions in the liver, heart, lungs and brain.

trace elements Substances that occur in very small quantities in in the body but are needed for its normal functioning.

tyramine A substance found in chocolate, mature cheeses, red wine, smoked fish products, brewer's yeast and MSG (monosodium glutamate) among other things. It causes migraine and other food intolerance reactions in susceptible people. It also raises blood pressure.

Further reading

CHILDREN AND EATING

Anorexia and Bulimia, Alexander Schauss Ph.D. and Carolyn Costin M.A. M.F.C.C., Keats Publishing, 1997

The Complete Baby and Toddler Meal Planner, Annabel Karmel, Ebury Press

The Hyperactive Child, Belinda Barnes and Irene Colquhoun, Thorson's, 1986

FOOD FOR HEALTH

Allergy and Intolerance, G. Lewith, J. Kenyon and D. Dowson, Martin Press, 1992

Balancing Hormones Naturally, Kate Neil. I.O.N. Press, 1994

Better Health Through Natural Healing, Ross Trattler, Thorson's, 1987

A Cancer Therapy, Max Gerson M.D., Gerson Institute, 1986

Encyclopaedia of Natural Medicine, Michael Murray and Joseph Pizzorno, Macdonald & Co., 1992

Food and Healing, Annemarie Colbin, Ballantine Books, 1983

Foods to Heal, Barry Fox, St Martin's, 1996

Living Food, Patrick Holford, Thorson's, 1994.

Natural Life Extension, Leon Chaitow, Thorson's, 1992

Nutritional Medicine, Dr. Stephen Davies and Dr. Alan Stewart, Pan Books, 1987

NUTRITION

Dietary Reference Values for Food Energy and Nutrients for the United Kingdom, HMSO, 1991

Encyclopaedia of Nutritional Supplements, Michael T. Murray, Prima, 1996

Essential Nutrients in Supplements, European Health Products Manufacturers' Association, 1995

Fats that Heal, Fats that Kill, Udo Erasmus, Alive Books, 1993

Food Science, Nutrition and Health, Brian A Fox and Allan G Cameron, E. Arnold, 1995

The Food System – A Guide, Geoff Tansey and Tony Worsley, Earth Scan, 1995

The New Nutrition, Dr. Michael Colgan, Apple Publishing, 1995

Nutrition and Evolution, Michael Crawford and David Marsh, Airlift, 1995

Toxemia: The Basic Cause of Disease, John H. Tilden M.D., Natural Hygiene Press, 1982

Thorsons Complete Guide to Vitamins and Minerals, Leonard Mervyn, Thorsons

The Antioxidant Health Plan, Dr. Robert Youngson, Thorson's, 1994

The Antioxidants, Richard A. Passwater Ph.D., Keats Publishing, 1985

Aspartame (NutraSweet): Is It Safe? H. J. Roberts M.D., Charles Press, 1990

Raw Energy Recipes, Leslie and Susannah Kenton, Century, 1985

The Super Supplements Bible, Dr. Michael E Rosenbaum and Dominick Bosco, Thorson's, 1988.

The Biogenic Diet, Leslie Kenton, Arrow Books, 1987.

The Principles of Nutritional Therapy, Linda Lazarides, Thorson's, 1996

Useful addresses

British Nutrition Foundation
High Holborn House
52-4 High Holborn
London WC1V 6RQ
Tel. (0171) 404 6504

Council for Nutrition Education and Therapy (CNEAT)
1 The Close Halton,
Aylesbury, Bucks
HP22 5NJ

Digestive Diseases Foundation
PO Box 251
Edgware
Middlesex HA8 6HG
Tel. (0171) 486 0341

Foresight (the Association for Preconceptual Care)
28 The Paddock
Godalming
Surrey GU7 1XD
Tel. (01483) 427839

The Hyperactive Children's Support Group
Mayfield House
Yapton Road, Barnham
West Sussex PO22 0BJ
Tel. 01903 725182

Institute for Optimum Nutrition (ION)
Blades Court
Deodar Road
London SW15 2NU
Tel. (0181) 877 9993

The Society for Promotion of Nutritional Therapy (SPNT)
PO Box 47
Heathfield
East Sussex TN21 8ZX
Tel. (01825) 872921
E-mail and Internet:
100045.255@compuserve.com

The Soil Association
Bristol House
40-56 Victoria Street
Bristol BS1 6BY
Tel. (0117) 9290661

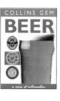

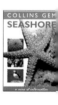

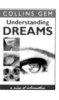